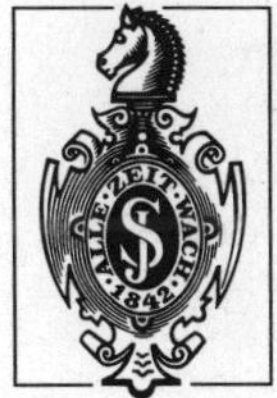

UICC International Union Against Cancer
Union Internationale Contre le Cancer

TNM Supplement 1993

A Commentary on Uniform Use

Edited by
P. Hermanek, D. E. Henson
R. V. P. Hutter, L. H. Sobin

With 26 Figures

Springer-Verlag
Berlin Heidelberg New York
London Paris Tokyo
Hong Kong Barcelona
Budapest

UICC
3, rue du Conseil-Général, CH–1205 Geneva, Switzerland

Editors:

Professor Dr. P. Hermanek
Vorstand der Abteilung für Klinische Pathologie i. R.
Chirurgische Universitätsklinik Erlangen
Maximiliansplatz, 91054 Erlangen, FRG

Dr. D. E. Henson
Early Detection Branch, Division of Cancer Prevention and Control
National Cancer Institute, Bethesda, MD 20892, USA

Dr. R. V. P. Hutter
Clinical Professor of Pathology
University of Medicine and Dentistry
New Jersey Medical School, Newark, NJ
Department of Pathology, Saint Barnabas Medical Center
Old Short Hills Road, Livingston, NJ 07039, USA

Dr. L. H. Sobin
Professor of Pathology
Uniformed Services University of the Health Sciences
Bethesda, MD, USA
Division of Gastrointestinal Pathology
Armed Forces Institute of Pathology, Washington, DC 20306, USA

ISBN 3-540-56556-6 Springer-Verlag Berlin Heidelberg New York
ISBN 0-387-56556-6 Springer-Verlag New York Berlin Heidelberg

Library of Congress Cataloging-in-Publication Data
TNM supplement 1993: a commentary on uniform use/edited by P. Hermanek ... [et al.]. p. cm. At head of title:
UICC. "Complement the 4th edition of the TNM classification ..." – -Preface. Includes bibliographical references
and index.
ISBN 3-540-56556-6. –
ISBN 0-387-56556-6
1. Tumors-Classification.   I. Hermanek, Paul.   II. International Union against Cancer.   III. TNM classification of
malignant tumours. RC258.T583   1992 Suppl. 616.99'4'0012–dc20   93-10973-CIP

Typesetting: Appl, Wemding
21/3145-5 4 3 2 1 0 – Printed on acid-free paper

Preface

The fourth edition of the *TNM Classification* was published in 1987,[1] and a revision in 1992.[2] It was the result of efforts by all national TNM Committees towards a worldwide uniform classification. The classification criteria are identical with the fourth edition of the *Manual for Staging of Cancer* of the American Joint Committee on Cancer (AJCC).[3] Although the classification has found wide acceptance, some workers have pointed out that individual definitions and rules for staging are not sufficiently detailed. This can lead to inconsistent application of the classification, the antithesis of standardization. This source of differences in interpretation applies not only to the classification of individual organs but also to the general rules of the system, especially to the definitions of the requirements for the pathological classification (pT, pN). These are specified only for carcinoma of the breast; for other sites, reference must be made back to the general rules, which can lead to variable interpretations.

The TNM Project Committee of the UICC has addressed this problem and collected and considered the criticisms and suggestions from the national TNM Committees as well as from cancer registries, oncological associations and individual users. The result was the decision to complement the 4th edition of the *TNM Classification*[1,2,3] with the publication of a *TNM Supplement* containing recommendations for the uniform use of TNM.

In the two chapters of "Explanatory Notes", the definitions of anatomical sites/subsites, regional lymph nodes and T, N and M categories that are generic or ambiguous are spelled out in a more precise manner. The minimum requirements for the pathological classification of individual tumour sites and entities are then detailed in the third chapter on "Site – Specific Recommendations for pT and pN".

---

[1] UICC (1987) TNM classification of malignant tumours, 4th edn (Hermanek P, Sobin LH, eds). Springer, Berlin Heidelberg New York

[2] UICC (1992) TNM classification of Malignant tumours, 4th edn, 2nd revision (Hermanek P, Sobin LH, eds). Springer, Berlin Heidelberg New York

[3] AJCC (1992) Manual for Staging of Cancer, 4th edn (Beahrs OH, Henson DE, Hutter RVP, Kennedy BJ, eds). Lippincott, Philadelphia

The UICC TNM Project Committee has reviewed several recommended changes and amendments for the *TNM Classification*. These are explained in the fourth and fifth chapters, on "Proposals for New Classifications" and "Optional Proposals for Testing New Telescopic Ramifications". Where data exist to support these recommendations we have included relevant references; where they do not, the proposals are based on anecdotal experience and/or general considerations. The UICC TNM Project Committee is of the opinion that these changes should be tested in the coming years. Consequently, several proposals for modification of the TNM system are contained in this *Supplement*. These are based on the principle of ramification, i. e. the T, N and M categories of the 4th edition remain unchanged but optional subdivisions are given within specified categories. By classifying according to these subdivisions one can later compare and determine to what extent a change of the present categories improves the classification with respect to prognostic statements or with a view to the choice of treatment. At the same time, the basic structure of the 4th edition classification remains unchanged.

Furthermore, recommendations are given for the classification of new tumour sites and entities which have not yet been formally included in the TNM system.

The present stage grouping as defined in the *TNM Classification of Malignant Tumours,* 4th edition, is generally based on the anatomical extent of disease, as described by T, N and M or pT, pN and pM. For some tumour sites or entities, however, additional factors are included, namely:

Age	Thyroid
Grade	Soft tissue
	Bone
	Prostate
	Brain
Residual tumour	Nephroblastoma
	Neuroblastoma
	Paediatric soft tissue sarcoma

The TNM Project Committee of the UICC and the AJCC recognize that in addition to the anatomical extent of disease, assessed before and during initial treatment, the residual tumour status after treatment, i. e. the R (residual tumor) classification, as well as other non anatomical factors (e. g. host factors, biochemical markers, DNA analysis, oncogenes, oncogene products) may be important for assessing outcome. These prognostic factors other than TNM and R are currently under investigation; their importance for treatment planning, analysis of treatment and design of future clinical trials will increase. The UICC and the AJCC therefore plan to publish a compilation of prognostic factors in addition to TNM i 1994.

Institutions and physicians interested in the further development of the TNM system are encouraged to test the recommendations for ramification of the existing classifications and those for classification of new tumour sites and entities over the next years. Publications of both retrospective and prospective studies are desired. The TNM Project Committee would appreciate receiving relevant information and is available for further information and consultation.

August 1993

P. Hermanek, Erlangen
D. E. Henson, Bethesda, MD
R. V. P. Hutter, Livingston, NJ
L. H. Sobin, Washington, DC

Acknowledgements

The Editors have much pleasure in acknowledging the great help received from the members of the UICC TNM Committee, the national TNM Committees and the Surveillance, Epidemiology and End Results (SEER) Program of the National Cancer Institute (USA).

Financial support by the National Cancer Institute (USA) through grant CA 38193 is gratefully acknowledged.

The Editors wish to express their thanks to Mrs. Judith Wagner, Erlangen, Germany, for her help with the preparation of the manuscript.

Finally, the editors wish to thank Springer-Verlag and its staff for their speedy handling of the matter as well as for the excellent presentation of the publication.

Contents

Site-Specific Recommendations for pT and pN 49

Abbreviations

AJCC	American Joint Committee on Cancer
DSK-TNM	Deutschsprachiges TNM-Komitee (TNM Committee of the German-speaking countries)
ECC	Erlangen Cancer Center (Germany)
ERCRC	Erlangen Registry of Colo-Rectal Cancer (Germany)
FIGO	Fédération Internationale de Gynécologie et d'Obstetrique (International Federation of Gynaecology and Obstetrics)
ICC	Italian Committee for TNM Cancer Classification
IDS for CRC	International Documentation System for Colorectal Cancer
JJC	Japanese Joint Committee (National TNM Committee)
SEER	Surveillance, Epidemiology and End Results Program of the National Cancer Institute (USA)
SGCRC	German Study Group on Colo-Rectal Carcinoma
UICC	International Union Against Cancer

Note: The various T, N and M categories as well as the categories of optional classifications like R, L, V, G should be written as common arabic numerals, not as subscripts, e.g. T1 (not T_1) and N3 (not N_3). Stages are designated by Roman numerals.

Explanatory Notes
General

The General Rules of the TNM System[1,2]

General Rule No. 2

Two classifications are described for each site, namely:

a) Clinical classification (Pretreatment clinical classification), designated **TNM** (or cTNM). This is based on evidence acquired before treatment. Such evidence arises from physical examination, imaging, endoscopy, biopsy, surgical exploration and other relevant examinations.

b) Pathological classification (Postsurgical histopathological classification), designated **pTNM.** This is based on the evidence acquired before treatment, supplemented or modified by the additional evidence acquired from surgery and from pathological examination. The pathological assessment of the primary tumour (pT) entails a resection of the primary tumour or biopsy adequate to evaluate the highest pT category. The pathological assessment of the regional lymph nodes (pN) entails removal of nodes adequate to validate the absence of regional lymph node metastasis (pN0) and sufficient to evaluate the highest pN category. The pathological assessment of distant metastasis (pM) entails microscopic examination.

TNM is a dual system that includes a clinical (pretreatment) and a pathological (postsurgical histopathological) classification. It is imperative to differentiate between them since they are based on different methods of examination and serve different purposes. The clinical classification is designated TNM or cTNM; the pathological, pTNM. When TNM ist used without a prefix, it implies the clinical classification (cTNM). The requirements for pathological classification are described on p. 49.

---

[1] UICC (1992) TNM Classification of Malignant Tumours, 4th edn, 2nd revision (Hermanek P, Sobin LH, eds). Springer, Berlin Heidelberg New York, pp. 5–6.

[2] AJCC (1992) Manual for Staging of Cancer, 4th edn (Beahrs OH, Henson DE, Hutter RVP, Kennedy BJ, eds) Lippincott, Philadelphia, p. 6.

In general, the cTNM is the basis for the choice of treatment and the pTNM the basis for prognostic assessment. In addition, the pTNM may determine adjuvant treatment. Treatment based on cTNM may have an effect on end results. Comparison between cTNM and pTNM can also help in evaluating the accuracy of the clinical and imaging methods used to determine the cTNM. Therefore, it is important to retain the clinical *as well as* the pathological classification in the medical record.

A tumour is primarily described by the clinical classification before treatment or before the decision not to treat. In addition, a pathological classification is performed if specific requirements are met (see Chap. 3, p. 49). Therefore, for an individual patient there may be a clinical classification T2N1M0 and a pathological classification pT2pNXpMX. For final stage grouping clinical and pathological data may be combined when only partial information is available in both the pathological classification and the clinical classification. The example above is expressed as pT2cN1cM0. For further discussion on the meaning and application of X (e. g. NX, MX) see p. 7.

General Rule No. 3

After assigning T, N and M and/or pT, pN and pM categories, these may be grouped into stages. The TNM classification and stage grouping, once established, must remain unchanged in the medical records. The clinical stage is essential to select and evaluate therapy, while the pathological stage provides the most precise data to estimate prognosis and calculate end results.

The rule that the TNM classification, once established, must remain unchanged in the patient's record applies to the definitive TNM classification determined just before initiation of treatment or before making the decision not to treat. If, for instance, the initial classification T2N0M0 is made in one hospital and is later changed to T2N1M0 after the patient is referred to another centre where special imaging techniques are available, then the latter classification, based on a special examination, is considered the definitive one.

Following two surgical procedures for a single lesion, the pTNM classification should be a composite of the histological examination of the specimens from both operations.

Example. Initial endoscopic polypectomy of a carcinoma of the ascending colon is classified pT1pNXpMX; the subsequent right hemicolectomy contains two lymph nodes with tumour, and a suspicious metastatic focus in the liver, later found to be a haemangioma, is excised – the classification is pT0pN1pM0. The definitive pTNM classification consists of the results of both operative specimens – pT1pN1pM0 (stage III).

General Rule No. 4

> If there is doubt concerning the correct T, N or M category to which a particular case should be allotted, then the lower (i. e. less advanced) category should be chosen. This will also be reflected in the stage grouping.

Example. Sonography of the liver: suspicious but no definitive evidence of metastasis – M0 (not M1).

If there are different results from different methods, the classification should be based on the most reliable method of assessment.

Example. Colorectal carcinoma, preoperative examination of the liver: sonography, suspicious, but no evidence of metastasis; CT, evidence of metastasis. The results of CT determine the classification – M1. However, if CT were negative, the case would be classified M0.

General Rule No. 5

> In the case of multiple simultaneous tumours in one organ, the tumour with the highest T category should be classified and the multiplicity or the number of tumours should be indicated in parentheses, e. g. T2(m) or T2(5). In simultaneous bilateral cancers of paired organs, each tumour should be classified independently. In tumours of the thyroid, liver, ovary, nephroblastoma and neuroblastoma, multiplicity is a criterion of T classification.

The following rules apply to grossly recognizable multiple simultaneous carcinomas. They do not apply to one grossly detected tumour associated with multiple separate microscopic foci.

1. Multiple synchronous tumours in one organ may be:
   a) Multiple noninvasive tumours
   b) Multiple invasive tumours
   c) Multiple invasive tumours with associated carcinoma in situ
   d) A single invasive tumour with associated carcinoma in situ
   For (a) the multiplicity should be indicated by the suffix "(m)", e. g. Tis(m). For (b) and (c) the tumour with the highest T category is classified and the multiplicity or the number of invasive tumours is indicated in parentheses, e. g. T2(m) or T2(4). For (c) and (d) the presence of associated carcinoma in situ may be indicated by the suffix "(is)", e. g. T3(m,is) or T2(3,is) or T2(is).
2. For classification of multiple simultaneous tumours in "one organ", the definitions of one organ listed in Table 1 should be applied. The tumours at these sites with the highest T category should be classified and the multiplicity or the number of tumours should be indicated in parentheses, e. g. T2(m) or T2(5). Examples of sites for separate classification of two tumours are:

Table 1. Definition of "one organ" for the classification of multiple simultaneous primary tumours: the listed sites/subsites are considered as "one organ"

	ICD-O code
Lip	C00.0,1,2,6
Oral cavity	C00.3–5, C02.0–3, C03, C04, C05.0, C06
Oropharynx	C01, C05.1,2, C09, C10.0,2,3
Nasopharynx	C11
Hypopharynx	C12, C13
Larynx	C10.1, C32.0–2
Maxillary sinus	C31.0
Parotid gland	C07
Submandibular (submaxillary) gland	C08.0
Sublingual gland	C08.1
Thyroid[a]	C73
Oesophagus	C15
Stomach	C16
Small intestine	C17
Colon and rectum	C18–C20
Anal canal	C21.1,2
Liver[a]	C22
Gallbladder	C23
Extrahepatic bile ducts	C24.0
Ampulla of Vater	C24.1
Pancreas	C25
Lung	C34
Pleura	C38.4
Bones	C40, C41
Soft tissues, peripheral	C47, C49
Retroperitoneum	C48
Mediastinum	C38.1–3
Skin except eyelid, anal margin and perianal skin	C44.0,2–9
Eyelid	C44.1
Anal margin and perianal skin	C44,5
Breast	C50
Vulva	C51
Vagina	C52
Cervix uteri	C53
Corpus uteri	C54
Ovary[a]	C56
Penis	C60
Prostate	C61
Testis	C62
Scrotum	C63.2
Kidney	C64
Renal pelvis and ureter	C65, C66
Urinary bladder	C67
Urethra	C68.0
Conjunctiva	C69.0
Uvea	C69.3,4
Retina	C69.2
Orbit	C69.6
Lacrimal gland	C69.5
Brain	C70.0, C71

[a] In this organ multiplicity is a criterion of T classification.

- Oropharynx and hypopharynx
- Submandibular gland and parotid gland
- Urinary bladder and urethra (separate tumours)
- Skin carcinoma of eyelid and neck
   Examples for classification of the tumour with the highest T category and indication of multiplicity (m symbol) or numbers of tumours:
- Two separate tumours of the hypopharynx
- Carcinoma of the caecum and the transverse colon
- Skin carcinoma of the trunk and the arm
- Carcinoma of renal pelvis and ureter

3. If a new primary cancer is diagnosed within 2 months, this new cancer is considered synchronous (based on criteria used by the SEER Program of the National Cancer Institute, USA).

The TNM Clinical and Pathological Classifications

T/pT Classification

1. When size is a criterion for the T/pT category, it is a measurement of the *invasive* component. If in the breast, for example, there is a large in situ component (e. g. 4 cm) and a small invasive component (e. g. 0.5 cm), the tumour is coded for the invasive component only, i. e. pT1a.
2. Penetration or perforation of visceral serosa is a criterion for the T classification of some tumour sites, e. g. stomach, colon, rectum, gallbladder, lung, ovary. It may be confirmed by histological examinations of biopsies or resection specimens or by cytological examination of specimens obtained by scraping the serosa overlying the primary tumour (Zeng et al. 1992).
3. The microscopic presence of tumour in lymphatic vessels or veins does not qualify as local spread of tumour as defined by the T classification (except for liver and kidney).

   Example. In carcinoma of the uterine cervix, direct invasion beyond the myometrium of the uterine cervix qualifies as parametrial invasion with T2a/b, but not if based only on the discontinuous presence of tumour cells in lymphatics of the parametrium. The L and V symbols (TNM classification 1992, p. 10) can be used to record lymphatic and venous involvement.

4. Direct spread of tumour into an adjacent organ, e. g. the liver from a gastric primary, is recorded in the T/pT classification and is not considered a distant metastasis; in contrast to this, direct spread of the primary tumour into regional lymph nodes is classified as lymph node metastasis.
5. The very uncommon cases with *direct extension* into an *adjacent organ* or structure not mentioned in the T definitions are classified as the highest T category.

   Example. Liver carcinoma invading the gallbladder or stomach – T4.

6. Tumour spillage is considered a criterion in the T classification of ovarian tumours and in the pT classification of nephroblastoma. For all other tumours, tumour spillage does not affect the TNM classification, stage grouping or R classification.

Regional Lymph Nodes

1. Sometimes a tumour involves more than one site or subsite. In this case the regional lymph nodes are those of the involved sites or subsites.

   Example. Carcinoma of the oesophagus involving the upper thoracic portion and the cervical oesophagus: the regional lymph nodes are those for intrathoracic oesophagus, i. e. the mediastinal and perigastric nodes (excluding the coeliac nodes), as well as those for cervical oesophagus, i. e. the cervical nodes.

2. In rare cases, one finds no metastases in the regional lymph nodes, but only in lymph nodes which drain an adjacent organ *directly invaded* by the primary tumour. The lymph nodes of the invaded site are considered as those of the primary site for N classification.

   Example. Carcinoma of the sigmoid colon with direct extension into an adjacent small bowel loop: pericolic lymph nodes are tumour-free, but metastases are found in two mesenteric lymph nodes in the vicinity of the invaded small bowel – this is classified as pT4pN1M0 (stage III).

N/pN Classification

1. The clinical category N0 ("no regional lymph node metastasis") includes lymph nodes not clinically suspicious for metastases even if they are palpable or visualized with imaging techniques. The clinical category N1 ("regional lymph node metastasis") is used when there is sufficient clinical evidence, such as firmness, enlargement or imaging changes. The term "adenopathy" is not precise enough to indicate lymph node metastasis.

2. Invasion of lymphatic vessels (tumour cells in endothelium-lined canals, so-called lymphangiosis carcinomatosa or lymphangitic spread) in a distant organ is coded as pM1, e. g. lymphangitic spread in the lung from prostatic carcinoma.

3. A tumour nodule greater than 3 mm across in the connective tissue in the lymph drainage area of a primary tumour without histological evidence of residual lymph node in the nodule is classified in the N category as a regional lymph node metastasis. However, a tumour nodule of up to 3 mm is classified in the T category, i. e. discontinuous extension.

M Classification

1. Positive cytology from the peritoneal cavity based on laparoscopy or laparotomy before any other surgical procedure is classified M1, except in the ovary, where it is classified in the T category (Martin and Goellner 1986; Jaehne et al. 1989; Maruyama 1991; Warshaw 1991) (see p. 14).
2. Isolated tumour cells found in bone marrow are classified as distant metastases. However, these cases should be identified and analysed separately from other M1 cases (see p. 102).
3. In tumours of the gastrointestinal tract, multiple tumour foci in the mucosa or submucosa ("skip metastasis") are not considered in the TNM classification and should not be classified as distant metastasis. However, they should be distinguished from synchronous primary tumours, for example those with obvious mucosal origin; they are then categorized as multiple tumours, e. g. T2(m).

Who Is Responsible for TNM Coding?

Data for TNM are derived from a variety of sources, e. g. the examining physician, the radiologist, the endoscoping gastroenterologist, the operating surgeon and the histopathologist. The final TNM classification and/or stage grouping rest with a designated individual who has access to the most complete data.

The Significance of X

An X classification of an individual component of TNM or pTNM, e. g. TX or pNX, does not necessarily signify inadequate staging. The practical value of staging in the individual situation is to be considered, e. g. in patients with distant metastasis an effort to assess N is without clinical significance. In selected pT1 tumours of the colorectum, pNX may be the result of the correct decision to treat by endoscopic polypectomy or local excision. Also, experience shows that – at least in some sites, e. g. colorectum or anal canal – in T1/pT1 tumours of low grade the incidence of regional lymph node metastasis as well as of distant metastasis is exceptionally rare and therefore no supplementary efforts need be made to assess the N and M categories.

Stage Grouping

1. The term "stage" should be used only for combinations of T, N and M or pT, pN and pM categories. The expressions "T stage" and "N stage" should be avoided; it is correct to speak of T categories or N categories.

2. The stage can be determined exclusively according to the clinical classification (TNM), exclusively according to the pathological classification (pTNM) or based on a combination of clinical and pathological findings (e. g. pT, pN and M or pT, N and M or T, N and pM). If available, the pathological classifications are to be used for stage grouping.

   Examples
   - Pedunculated polyp of sigmoid colon discovered endoscopically, superficial biopsy: tubular adenoma with carcinoma in situ. Endoscopically, no suspicion of invasion. No regional lymph node or distant metastasis. Clinical classification – Tis N0M0.
     Endoscopic polypectomy: adenocarcinoma arising in a tubular adenoma invading the superficial stalk, with clear deep stalk. No further treatment. Pathological classification – pT1pNXpMX. Summarizing classification – pT1cN0cM0 or pT1N0M0, stage I. This is justified because experience shows that the incidence of regional lymph node metastasis and distant metastasis in pT1 is very rare.
   - Primary tumour of head and neck. Clinical diagnosis of regional lymph node metastasis by CT, no signs of distant metastasis. Treatment by surgical local excision of the primary tumour and radiotherapy of cervical lymph nodes. Clinical classification – T1N1M0. Pathological classification – pT1pNXpMX. Summarizing classification – pT1cN1cM0 or pT1N1M0, stage III.

3. In the assessment of distant metastases, the entire situation must be considered. If there is only a clinically determined M1 in an organ which could not be microscopically examined, this finding must be taken into consideration, even when there has been a simultaneous pM0 for another organ.

   Example. Colon carcinoma with multiple lung metastases (by radiography). Resection of the colon carcinoma because of stenosis – pT3pN2. Simultaneously, also local excision of areas suspicious for metastasis in liver, histologically found to be haemangioma. Final classification – pT3pN2M1, stage IV.

4. If T or N cannot be determined, stage grouping is only possible under the following circumstances:
   - Despite TX/pTX, stage grouping can be undertaken on the basis of N and M or pN and pM findings.

     Example. A firm head of pancreas with a grossly involved peripancreatic lymph node and no signs of distant metastasis at surgery – TXN1M0, stage III.

   - Despite NX/pNX, stage grouping can be undertaken when M/pM classification is possible.

     Example. A carcinoma of the pancreas with liver metastasis T1NXM1, stage IV. Cases with M1 or pM1 are classified as stage IV even in cases of T/pTX and N/pNX.

   - Despite NX/pNX, stage grouping is possible when a stage defined by a T category and M0 is provided.

     Example. Carcinoma of the oesophagus with invasion of trachea, regional lymph nodes not assessable, no signs of distant metastasis – T4NXM0, stage III.

– Cases of Tis (clinical classification based on biopsy) or pTis (pathological classification based on the examination of the resected lesion) are always classified as stage 0, even with NX/pNX and MX/pMX, because by definition no metastases can be present.

Residual Tumor (R) Classification

TNM and pTNM describe the anatomical extent of cancer in general without considering treatment. The residual tumour (R) classification deals with tumour status after treatment. It reflects the effects of treatment, influences further therapeutic procedures and is a strong predictor of prognosis (Figs. 1–3).

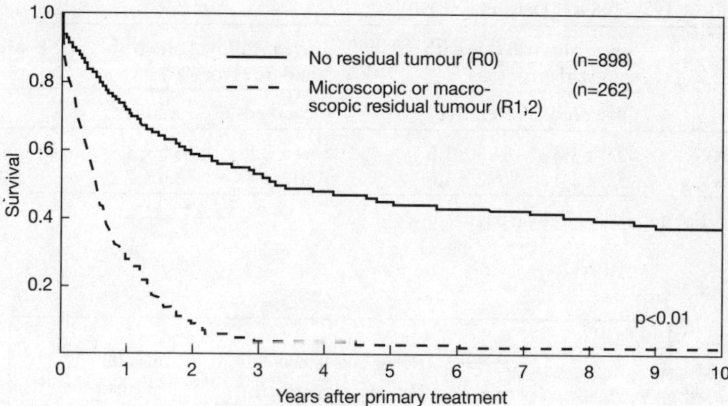

Fig. 1. Stomach carcinoma: observed and relative survival (Kaplan-Meier) in relation to the R classification, surgical mortality not excluded* (Department of Surgery, University of Erlangen, FRG, 1978–1989/31 December 1990)

	5-year survival rate with standard error (%)		10-year survival rate with standard error (%)		Median survival time (months)
	Observed	Relative	Observed	Relative	
R0	44.7 ± 2.2	54.9 ± 2.7	36.2 ± 3.6	57.9 ± 5.7	39.2
R1,2	2.8 ± 1.2	3.5 ± 1.4	2.4 ± 1.2	3.8 ± 1.9	6.4

* Note. The survival curves in the figure relate to observed survival calculated according to Kaplan-Meier without exclusion of surgical mortality. The figures for 5-year and 10-year survival are stated in the legend. Here also are added the relative (so-called age-corrected) survival rates as ratios of the observed to the expected survival rates. The latter were calculated from demographic data published regularly by the German Federal Office for Statistics and consider sex, age and period of observation.

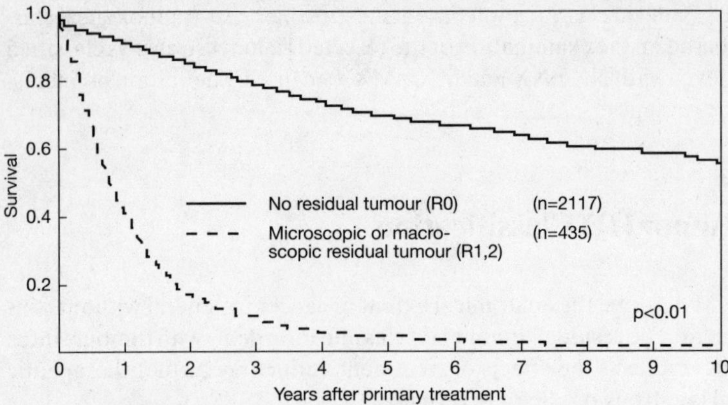

Fig. 2. Colorectal carcinoma: observed and relative survival (Kaplan-Meier) in relation to the R classification, surgical mortality not excluded* (Department of Surgery, University of Erlangen, FRG, 1978–1989/31 December 1990)

	5-year survival rate with standard error (%)		10-year survival rate with standard error (%)		Median survival time (months)
	Observed	Relative	Observed	Relative	
R0	69.9 ± 1.3	84.3 ± 1.6	56.4 ± 2.5	86.5 ± 3.8	undefined
R1,2	5.2 ± 1.4	6.2 ± 1.6	2.0 ± 1.4	3.0 ± 2.2	8.9

* For detail see Note on page 9.

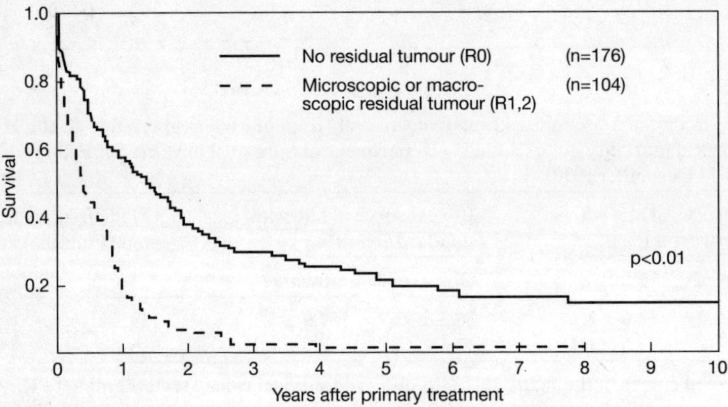

Fig. 3. Squamous cell carcinoma of the intrathoracic oesophagus: observed and relative survival (Kaplan-Meier) in relation to the R classification, surgical mortality not excluded* (Department of Surgery, University of Erlangen, FRG, 1978–1989/31 December 1990)

	5-year survival rate with standard error (%)		10-year survival rate with standard error (%)		Median survival time (months)
	Observed	Relative	Observed	Relative	
R0	21.1 ± 5.0	23.8 ± 5.7	13.8 ± 7.4	18.3 ± 9.9	16.3
R1,2	1.0 ± 1.0	1.1 ± 1.1	–	–	4.2

* For details see Note on page 9.

This R classification must be differentiated from the completely different Japanese R classification which classifies tumour resections according to the extent of lymph node dissection.

The Japanese Joint Comittee for TNM classification decided in 1993 to use the symbol D to classify the extent of lymph node dissection in place of R in the coming editions of their General Rules (Japanese Research Society for Gastric Cancer 1993) to avoid confusion with the Residual Tumor Classification of TNM.

In the R classification, not only is local-regional residual tumour to be taken into consideration, but also distant residual tumour in the form of remaining distant metastases. Figure 4 shows for colorectal carcinoma that prognosis is poor in patients with local-regional residual tumour only, as well as in those with distant residual tumour only and those with residual tumour in both sites.

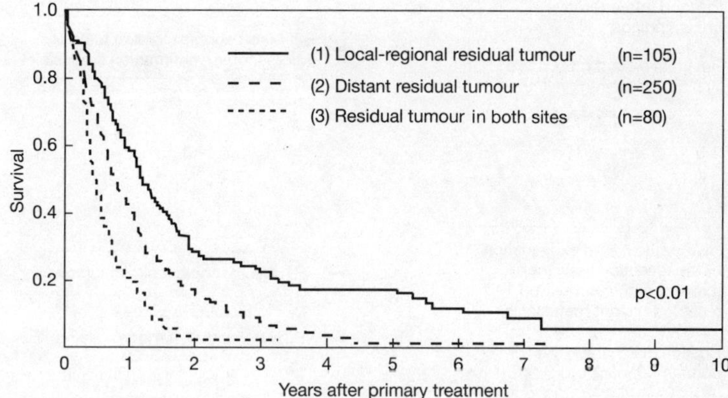

Fig. 4. Colorectal carcinoma with residual tumour: observed and relative survival (Kaplan-Meier) in relation to the site of residual tumour, surgical mortality not excluded* (Department of Surgery, University of Erlangen, FRG, 1978–1989/31 December 1990)

	5-year survival rate with standard error (%)		10-year survival rate with standard error (%)		Median survival time (months)
	Observed	Relative	Observed	Relative	
1	17.0 ± 4.3	20.8 ± 5.3	5.1 ± 3.6	6.5 ± 3.6	14.1
2	0.9 ± 0.9	1.1 ± 1.1	–	–	8.8
3	0	0	0	0	5.3

* For details see Note on page 9.

R0 corresponds to complete remission or resection for cure. It is appropriate for cases in which residual tumour cannot be detected by any diagnostic means. R0 classification, therefore, does not exclude nondetectable residual tumour which may give rise to tumour recurrence or metastasis during follow-up. R0, in fact, corresponds to *no detectable residual tumour* and is not identical to cure.

The R classification can be used following surgical treatment alone, after radiotherapy alone, after chemotherapy alone or following multimodal therapy. After nonsurgical treatment, the presence or absence of residual tumour is determined using clinical methods. Following surgical treatment, the R classification is possible through close cooperation between the surgeon and pathologist in a two-step process illustrated in Fig. 5.

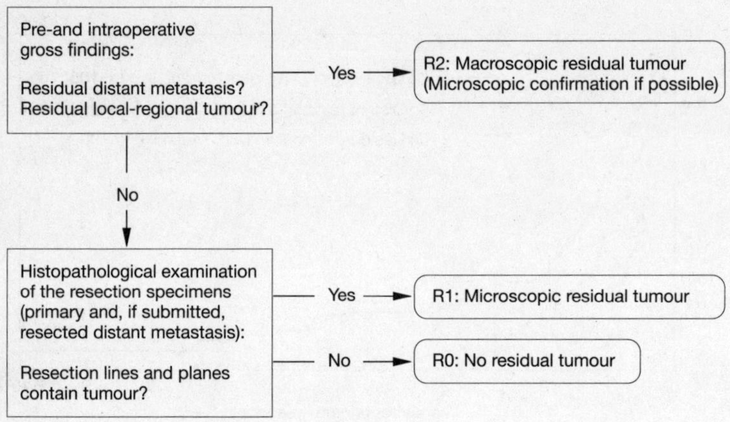

Fig. 5. R classification following surgery

In the R0 group there may be M0 cases as well as M1 cases. In the latter, not only the primary tumour and its lymphatic drainage but also the distant metastasis must be removed completely. Within the M1 group, there are statistically significant differences in relation to the R classification (Figs. 6, 7).

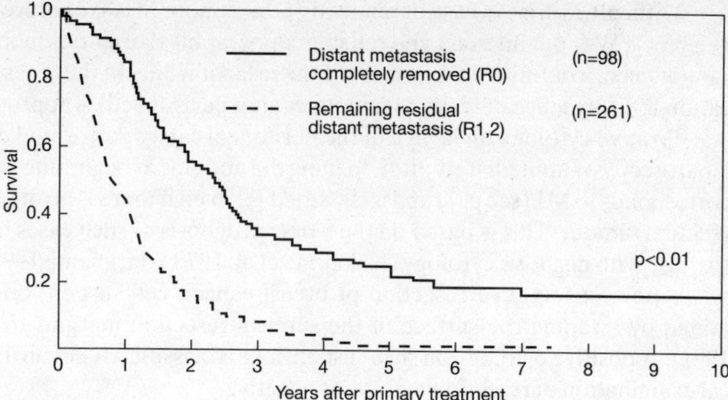

Fig. 6. Colorectal carcinoma with distant metastasis: observed and relative survival (Kaplan-Meier) in relation to the R classification, surgical mortality not excluded.* R1,2 includes remaining not resected metastasis as well as incompletely resected metastasis. (Department of Surgery, University of Erlangen, FRG, 1978–1989/31 December 1990)

	5-year survival rate with standard error (%)		10-year survival rate with standard error (%)		Median survival time (months)
	Observed	Relative	Observed	Relative	
R0	22.5 ± 4.8	26.0 ± 5.6	16.1 ± 10.4	22.5 ± 14.6	27.0
R1,2	0.8 ± 0.6	0.9 ± 0.9	–	–	8.9

* For details see Note on page 9.

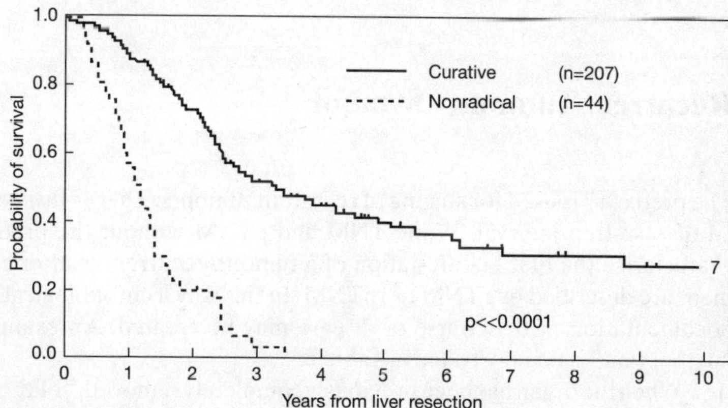

Fig. 7. Survival following resection of liver metastases. *Curative,* complete resection R0; *nonradical,* incomplete resection R1 or R2. (From Scheele et al. 1991)

In tumour resection specimens with formal lymphadenectomy the "marginal" lymph node is the one near the resection line that is most distant from the primary tumour. Involvement of such "marginal" or "apical" nodes does not influence the R classification.

Difficulties arise in case of removal of the tumour in two or more parts and not "en bloc". Without an exact and reliable topographical orientation the pathologist cannot make a definitive assessment of the resection line. In these cases the classification RX (presence of residual tumour cannot be assessed) is appropriate.

Positive cytology on lavage of the peritoneal cavity performed during staging laparoscopy or immediately after opening the abdomen (beginning of laparotomy) corresponds to M1 (see p. 7) and is classified R1 even if there is no other evidence of residual tumour. This is based on the worse prognosis of such cases in comparison to those with negative cytology (Nakajima et al. 1978; Maruyama 1991).

After conservative resection of breast cancer, cell suspensions may be obtained by scraping the surface of the surgical resection margins (Veronesi et al. 1991). A positive cytology on such suspensions is classified R1 even if the histological examination of resection margins is negative.

L Classification

Lymphatic vessels include those within and at the margins of the primary tumour as well as afferent and efferent lymphatics further away. Invasion of small lymphatic vessels requires the demonstration of tumour cells (single or groups) within channels which are unequivocally lined with endothelium. The finding of spaces around tumour nests caused by shrinkage during embedding should not be mistaken for lymphatic invasion.

Recurrent Tumour, r Symbol

The prefix "r" is used for staging of recurrent tumours. There *must* be a documented disease-free interval. While TNM and pTNM without the prefix "r" always characterize the first manifestation of a tumour, recurrences after curative treatment are described by rTNM or rpTNM. In this way a chronological TNM/pTNM documentation of the course of disease may be created. An example of such a "pathogram" is demonstrated in Table 2.

When the organ has been previously completely removed, "rTX" is used except if there is recurrence at the incision site or suture line anastomotic site. In these cases an "rT" category may be used that best describes the recurrence at the primary site.

Examples
1. Previous radical mastectomy, without remaining local-regional residual tumour. Local recurrence in the scar, 1.5 cm in greatest dimension – rT1c.
2. Previous total gastrectomy, without remaining local-regional residual tumour. Local recurrence at the oesophagojejunostomy involving mucosa, submucosa, muscularis propria and perimuscular tissue – rT3.

Table 2. "Pathogram" of a patient with rectal carcinoma

Date	Treatment	TNM/pTNM/R
April 1982	Complete local excision (perianal disc excision)	T1N0M0 pT1pN0pMX/R0
July 1982 October 1982 January 1983 April 1983 July 1983	–	rT0N0M0
October 1983	Low anterior resection	rT1N0M0 rpT2pN1pMX/R0
January 1984 April 1984 July 1984	–	rT0N0M0
October 1984	Liver resection	rT0N0M1 (Liver) rT0N0pM1/R0
January 1985	–	rT0N0M0
Last contact January 1990	–	rT0N0M0

Patients with Unknown Primary Tumour

In patients with an unknown primary tumour, the staging is based on the regional lymph node and/or distant metastasis status. The category T0 is applied to the primary tumour.

Example. Metastatic melanoma in cervical lymph node less than 3 cm in greatest dimension without primary or other metastasis – T0N1M0, stage III.

Staging of Tumours for Which No TNM Classification Is Provided

Staging according to the rules of the SEER Program is recommended if no TNM classification is provided. Staging is based on the concept of local, regional and distant

- In situ (noninvasive, intraepithelial)
- Localized (confined to the organ of origin)
- Regional, direct extension
- Regional, lymph nodes
- Regional, direct extension and lymph nodes
- Distant, direct extension or metastasis
- Distant, lymph nodes

Histopathological Grading

Histopathological grading of tumours of the same histological type is performed to provide some indication of their aggressiveness, which may in turn relate to prognosis or treatment. Grading should follow the recommendations of the WHO International Histological Classification of Tumours.

For most sites, histopathological grading consists of four grades:

G1   Well differentiated
G2   Moderately differentiated
G3   Poorly differentiated
G4   Undifferentiated

In the event that there are different degrees of differentiation in a tumour, one should assign the tumour to the least favourable grade of G1–G3.

Example. Partially well differentiated, partially moderately differentiated adenocarcinoma of the colon – G2.

G1 and G2 may be grouped together as low grade (G1–2), G3 and G4 as high grade (G3–4). In some tumour sites, no differentiation is made between G3 and G4 and therefore the category G3–4 is used. This is valid for carcinoma of the uterine corpus, ovary, penis, prostate, kidney, renal pelvis, ureter, urinary bladder and urethra.

Only three grades (G1–G3) are used for malignant melanoma of the conjunctiva and uvea.

In carcinoma of the thyroid, pleural mesothelioma, malignant melanoma of the skin and of the eyelids, retinoblastoma, malignant testicular tumours, nephroblastoma and neuroblastoma, grading is not applicable.

In undifferentiated carcinomas of the oesophagus, stomach, gallbladder, pancreas and colorectum, the category G4 is appropriate. By definition, an adenocarcinoma of these organs can be classified only as G1, G2 or G3. When, in an adenocarcinoma of these organs, there are undifferentiated areas next to areas with glandular differentiation, the tumour is classified as a poorly differentiated adenocarcinoma, because the diagnosis "undifferentiated carcinoma" is reserved only for those tumours with no specific differentiation at all. The same applies for squamous cell carcinoma with undifferentiated areas.

In some sites the WHO classification lists no "undifferentiated carcinoma" as a specific tumour type, e. g. in lung and breast. In those cases the category G4 is not applied (Henson et al. 1991).

In the absence of an assigned grade the following can be considered G4:

– Undifferentiated carcinoma (where provided)
– Small cell carcinoma (any site)
– Large cell carcinoma of lung
– Ewing sarcoma of bone and soft tissue
– Rhabdomyosarcoma of soft tissue

In grading, different methods may be appropriate for the various tumour entities (type and site). For example, in gastrointestinal adenocarcinomas the growing edge of a tumour should not be assessed as it may appear to be of high grade (Jass and Sobin 1989); in contrast grading which considers the histologically invasive edge is appropriate for predicting the prognosis of oral squamous cell carcinoma (Bryne et al. 1989).

Grading is generally performed by a combined evaluation of various histological and cytological features, including similarity to tissue of origin, cell arrangement, cellularity, differentiation, cellular and nuclear pleomorphism, mitotic activity, necrosis and others. Grading is a subjective procedure which requires considerable experience by the pathologist. To reduce individual veriability and to increase reproducibility of grading semiquantitative methods have been proposed. Various morphological parameters have been scored from 1 to 3 or 1 to 4, and the scores for each variable added into a total malignancy score for each tumour. A high malignancy score suggests a poorly differentiated tumour. Such grading systems have been published for breast carcinoma (Bloom and Richardson 1957; Schnürch et al. 1989), soft tissue sarcomas (Coindre et al. 1987; Enzinger and Weiss 1988), prostate carcinoma (Gleason and VACURG 1977; Müller et al. 1980) and oral squamous cell carcinoma (Anneroth and Hansen 1984; Anneroth et al. 1987; Bryne et al. 1989). The pathologist should indicate the grading system used in his report.

References

Anneroth G, Hansen LS (1984) A methodologic study of histologic classification and grading of malignancy in oral squamous cell carcinoma. Scand J Dent Res 92: 448–468

Anneroth G, Batsakis J, Luna M (1987) Review of the literature and a recommended system of malignancy grading in oral squamous cell carcinoma. Scand J Dent Res 95: 229–249

Bloom HJG, Richardson WW (1957) Histologic grading and prognosis in breast cancer. Br J Cancer 11: 359–377

Bryne M, Koppang HS, Lilleng R, Stene T, Bang G, Dabelsteen E (1989) New malignancy grading is a better prognostic indicator than Broders' grading in oral squamous cell carcinomas. J Oral Pathol Med 18: 432–437

Coindre JM, Trojani M, Contesso G et al. (1986) Reproducibility of a histopathological grading system for adult tissue sarcoma. Cancer 58: 306–309

Enzinger FM, Weiss SW (1988) Soft tissue tumors, 2nd edn, Mosby, St. Louis

Gleason DF, Veterans Administration Cooperative Urological Research Group (VACURG) (1977) Histologic grading and clinical staging of prostatic carcinoma. In: Tannenbaum M (ed) Urologic pathology: the prostate. Lea and Febiger, Philadelphia

Henson DE, Ries L, Freedman LS, Carriaga M (1991) Relationship among outcome, stage of disease, and histologic grade for 22 616 cases of breast cancer. Cancer 68: 2142–2149

Jaehne J, Meyer HJ, Soudah B, Maschek H, Pichlmayr R (1989) Peritoneal lavage in gastric carcinoma. Dig Surg 6: 26–28

Japanese Research Society for Gastric Cancer (1993) The general rules for gastric cancer study. 12th ed. (in Japanese). Kanahare Public Co Ltd, Tokyo

Jass JR, Sobin LH (1989) Histological typing of intestinal tumours, 2nd edn. WHO International Histological Classification of Tumours. Springer, Berlin Heidelberg New York

Martin JK Jr, Goellner JR (1986) Abdominal fluid cytology in patients with gastrointestinal malignant lesions. Mayo Clin Proc 61: 467–471

Maruyama K (1991) Diagnosis of invisible peritoneal metastasis: cytologic examination by peritoneal lavage. In: Cordiano C, de Manzoni G (eds) Staging and treatment of gastric cancer. Piccin Nuova Libraria, Padua, pp 180–181

Müller HA, Alternähr E, Böcking A, Dhom G, Faul P, Göttinger H, Helpap B, Hohbach C, Kastendieck H, Leistenschneider G (1980) Über Klassifikation und Grading des Prostatacarcinomas. Verh Dtsch Ges Path 64: 609–611

Nakajima T, Harashima S, Hirata M, Kajitani T (1978) Prognostic and therapeutic values of peritoneal cytology in gastric cancer. Acta Cytol 22: 225–229

Scheele J, Stangl R, Altendorf-Hofmann A, Gall FP (1990) Indicators of prognosis after hepatic resection for colorectal secondaries. Surgery 110: 13–29

Schnürch HG, Lange C, Bender HG (1989) Vier histopathologische Differenzierungsgrade beim Mammakarzinom? Pathologe 10: 39–42

SEER Program (1992) Code manual. Revised edition June 1992 (Cunningham J, Ries L, Hankey B, Seiffert J, Lyles B, Shambaugh E, Percy C, van Holten V, eds) NIH Publication No 92–1999. National Cancer Institute, Bethesda

Veronesi U, Farante G, Galimberti V, Greco M, Luini A, Sacchini V, Andreola S, Leoni F, Ménard S, Ronco M, Colnaghi MI (1991) Evaluation of resection margins after breast conservative surgery with monoclonal antibodies. Eur J Surg Oncol 17: 338–341

Warshaw AL (1991) Implications of peritoneal cytology for staging of early pancreatic cancer. Am J Surg 161: 26–30

Zeng Z, Cohen AM, Hajdu S, Sternberg SS, Sigurdson ER, Enker W (1992) Serosal cytologic study to determine free mesothelial penetration by intraperitoneal colon cancer. Cancer 70: 737–740

Explanatory Notes
Specific Anatomical Sites

Head and Neck Tumours

General

Anatomy

A uniform topographic terminology should be used for classification, and the sites, subsites, adjacent sites and adjacent structures should be clearly distinguished.

Sites and Subsites

Sites	Subsites
Lip (C00)[1]	1. External upper lip (vermilion border) (C00.0)
	2. External lower lip (vermilion border) (C00.1)
	3. Commissures (C00.6)
Oral Cavity	1. Buccal mucosa
	i) Mucosa of upper and lower lips (C00.3,4)
	ii) Cheek mucosa (C06.0)
	iii) Retromolar areas (C06.2)
	iv) Buccoalveolar sulci, upper and lower (vestibule of moth) (C06.1)
	2. Upper alveolus and gingiva (upper gum) (C03.0)
	3. Lower alveolus and gingiva (lower gum) (C03.1)
	4. Hard palate (C05.0)
	5. Tongue
	i) Dorsal surface and lateral borders anterior to vallate papillae (anterior two-thirds) (C02.0,1)
	ii) Inferior (ventral) surface (C02.2)
	6. Floor of mouth (C04)
Oropharynx (C10)	1. Anterior wall (glossoepiglottic area)
	i) Base of tongue (posterior to the vallate) papillae or posterior third) (C01)
	ii) Vallecula (C10.0)

---

[1] Note. Topography code of the WHO International Classification of Diseases for Oncology (ICD-O), 2nd ed (C Percy, V van Holten, C Muir). WHO, Geneva (1990)

2. Lateral wall (C10.2)
   i)   Tonsil (C09.9)
   ii) Tonsillar fossa (C09.0) and tonsillar
       (faucial) pillars (C09.1)
   iii) Glossotonsillar sulci (tonsillar pillars) (C09.1)
3. Posterior wall (C10.3)
4. Superior wall
   i)   Inferior surface of soft palate (C05.1)
   ii) Uvula (C05.2)

Nasopharynx (C11)

1. Posterosuperior wall: extends from the level of the junction of the hard and soft palates to the base of the skull (C11.0,1)
2. Lateral wall: including the fossa of Rosenmüller (C11.2)
3. Inferior wall: consists of the superior surface of the soft palate (C11.3)

Note. The margin of the choanal orifices, including the posterior margin of the nasal septum, is included with the nasal fossa.

Hypopharynx (C12, C13)

1. Pharyngo-oesophageal junction (postcricoid area) (C13.0): extends from the level of the arytenoid cartilages and connecting folds to the inferior border of the cricoid cartilage
2. Piriform sinus (C12.9): extends from the pharyngo-epiglottic fold to the upper end of the oesophagus. It is bounded laterally by the thyroid cartilage and medially by the hypopharyngeal surface of the aryepiglottic fold (13.1) and the arytenoid and cricoid cartilages
3. Posterior pharyngeal wall (13.2): extends from the level of the floor of the vallecula to the level of the inferior border of the cricoid cartilage

Supraglottis (C32.1)

   i)   Suprahyoid epiglottis (including tip, lingual [anterior] [C10.1] and laryngeal surfaces)
   ii) Aryepiglottic fold, laryngeal aspect
   iii) Arytenoid
   iv) Infrahyoid epiglottis
   v) Ventricular bands (false cords)

Glottis (C32.0)

   i)   Vocal cords
   ii) Anterior commissure
   iii) Posterior commissure

Subglottis (C32.2)
Maxillary Sinus (C31.0)
Parotid Gland (C07.9)
Submandibular Gland (C08.0)
Sublingual Gland (C08.1)
Thyroid Gland (C73.9)

Tumours Involving Two Sites

Tumours involving two anatomical sites are classified according to the site in which the greater part of the tumour is located. In invasive tumours with an associated carcinoma in situ only the invasive component is considered.

Example. Carcinoma with two-thirds in the hypopharynx and one-third in the supraglottis is classified as hypopharynx carcinoma.

Adjacent Structures

Adjacent structures are structures which can be invaded by a tumour only in the case of extensive deep invasion, e. g. extension of a glottis carcinoma through thyroid cartilage into soft tissues of the neck or extension of a carcinoma of the maxillary sinus through the floor or medial wall of orbit into the orbit.

Extension to Adjacent Sites
(Proposal Steiner and Ambrosch 1993 and DSK-TNM)

In tumours extending to an adjacent site, differentiation between superficial extension and deep extension is necessary. In superficial extension the involvement is limited to the mucosa, in deep extension muscles, bones or other deeper structures are invaded.

Superficial extension to adjacent sites is not considered as invasion of adjacent structures (T4).

Example. A tumour extending from the oropharynx to nasopharynx or hypopharynx or to oral cavity and limited to the mucosa (without invasion of muscles, bones or other deeper structures) is classified only according to size. The involvement of nasopharynx or hypopharynx or oral cavity is not considered invasion of adjacent structures provided that the tumour is limited to the mucosa.

Deep extension to an adjacent site can be the result of vertical invasion of adjacent structures (see above) or the result of horizontal spread *not* limited to the mucosa but also involving muscles or bones. It is classified as invasion of adjacent structures (T4).

Example. Carcinoma of the hypopharynx involving the submucosa and muscle layer of the oesophagus, with or without mucosal involvement.

Regional Lymph Nodes

According to the *TNM Atlas* the cervical nodes include the following node groups (Fig. 8):

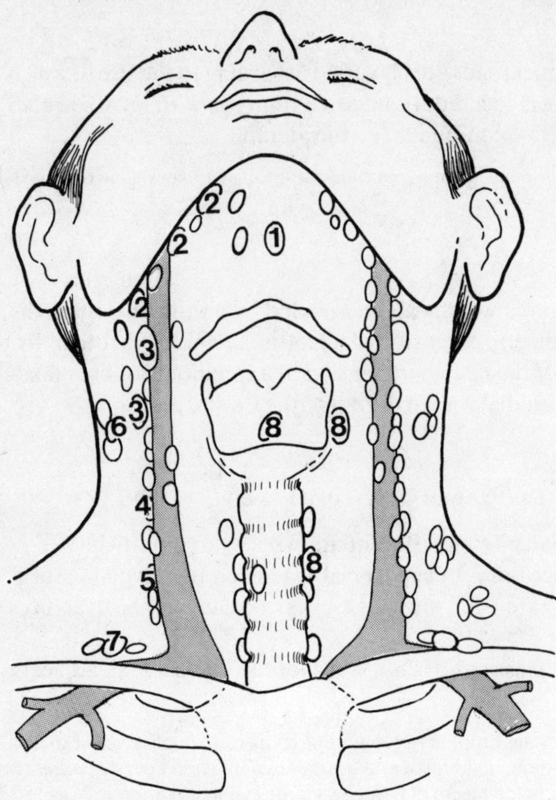

Fig. 8. Cervical lymph node groups. (From TNM Atlas 1992)

1. Submental nodes
2. Submandibular nodes (syn. submaxillary nodes)
3. Cranial jugular (deep cervical) nodes
4. Medial jugular (deep cervical) nodes
5. Caudal jugular (deep cervical) nodes
6. Dorsal cervical (superficial cervical) nodes along the accessory nerve
7. Supraclavicular nodes
8. Prelaryngeal and paratracheal (syn. anterior cervical) nodes
9. Retropharyngeal nodes
10. Parotid nodes
11. Buccal nodes (syn. facial nodes)
12. Retroauricular (syn. mastoid, posterior auricular) and occipital nodes

In 1991, a standardized neck dissection terminology was published by a Committee for Head and Neck Surgery and Oncology of the American Academy for Oto-laryngology – Head and Neck Surgery (Robbins et al. 1991). In October 1992, at an international symposium in Göttingen, Germany, this terminology was accepted by representatives of various European cancer centres (Villejuif, Milan, Amsterdam). We support the use of this terminology (Robbins et al. 1991). The lymph node groups 1–8 are defined as follows:

1. *Submental group:*
   Lymph nodes within the triangular boundary of the anterior belly of the digastric muscle and the hyoid bone.
2. *Submandibular group:*
   Lymph nodes within the boundaries of the anterior and posterior bellies of the digastric muscle and the body of the mandible.
3. *Upper jugular group:*
   Lymph nodes located around the upper third of the internal jugular vein and adjacent spinal accessory nerve, extending from the level of the carotid bifurcation (surgical landmark) or hyoid bone (clinical landmark) to the skull base. The posterior boundary is the posterior border of the sternocleidomastoid muscle, and the anterior boundary is the lateral border of the sternohyoid muscle. This group includes the jugulodigastric node, which is the most cranial jugular node.
4. *Middle jugular group:*
   Lymph nodes located around the middle third of the internal jugular vein, extending from the carotid bifurcation superiorly to the omohyoid muscle (surgical landmark) or cricothyroid notch (clinical landmark) inferiorly. The posterior boundary is the posterior border of the sternocleidomastoid muscle, and the anterior boundary is the lateral border of the sternohyoid muscle. This group includes the juguloomohyoid node located between omohyoid muscle and internal jugular vein.
5. *Lower jugular group:*
   Lymph nodes located around the lower third of the internal jugular vein, extending from the omohyoid muscle superiorly to the clavicle inferiorly. The posterior boundary is the posterior border of the sternocleidomastoid muscle, and the anterior boundary is the lateral border of the sternohyoid muscle.
6. *Dorsal cervical nodes along the accessory nerve and*
7. *Supraclavicular nodes:*
   The two groups are combined and called the *"Posterior triangle group":* This comprises predominantly the lymph nodes located along the lower half of the spinal accessory nerve and the transverse cervical artery. The supraclavicular nodes are also included. The posterior boundary is the anterior border of the trapezius muscle, the anterior boundary is the posterior border of the sternocleidomastoid muscle, and the inferior border is the clavicle.
8. *Anterior compartment group:*
   Lymph nodes surrounding the midline visceral structures of the neck, extending from the level of the hyoid bone superiorly to the suprasternal notch inferiorly. On each side, the lateral boundary is the medial border of the carotid sheath. Located within this compartment are the perithyroidal lymph nodes, paratracheal lymph nodes, lymph nodes along the recurrent laryngeal nerves and precricoid lymph nodes. See also p. 24 and Fig. 9.

The lymph node groups 1–8 may be grouped into levels:

Level (Robbins et al. 1991)	Lymph node group number	Lymph node terminology TNM Atlas (1992)	Robbins et al. (1991)
I	1	Submental nodes	Submental group
	2	Submandibular nodes	Submandibular group
II	3	Cranial jugular nodes	Upper jugular group
III	4	Medial jugular nodes	Middle jugular group
IV	5	Caudal jugular nodes	Lower jugular group
V	6	Dorsal cervical nodes along the accessory nerve	Posterior triangle group
	7	Supraclavicular nodes	
VI	8	Prelaryngeal and para-tracheal nodes	Anterior compartment group

The *parotid nodes* (10) may be subdivided into superficial (in front of tragus on top of parotid fascia) and deep parotid nodes. The latter are located underneath the parotid fascia and include intraglandular nodes directly in parotid gland. The preauricular and infraauricular (infra- or subparotid) nodes are assigned to the parotid nodes.

The *buccal (facial) nodes* (11) include the buccinator nodes located deep on buccinator muscle, the nasolabial nodes located underneath nasolabial groove, the molar nodes located in the surface of cheek and the mandibular nodes located outside the lower jaw.

For *thyroid surgery*, a distinction between a central and a lateral compartment is of interest for treatment planning (Dralle 1992). The central compartment includes groups 1, 2 and 8; the lateral compartment groups 3–7.

Node group 8 (prelaryngeal and paratracheal nodes) may be further subdivided as follows (Fig. 9):

– 8a: cranial paratracheal (suprathyroidal)
– 8b: thyroidal (perithyroidal)
– 8c: caudal paratracheal (infrathyroidal, lateral tracheal)
– 8d: prelaryngeal
– 8e: pretracheal near the thyroid isthmus (delphian)

The regional lymph nodes for thyroid include the *upper mediastinal lymph nodes*, which may be subdivided into tracheo-oesophageal (posterior mediastinal) and upper anterior mediastinal nodes. Cervical and mediastinal lymph nodes are not divided by a fascia; the left brachiocephalic vein is considered as the boundary (Dralle 1992).

N Classification

Size of Lymph Nodes: In advanced lymphatic spread, one often finds perinodal tumour and the confluence of several lymph node metastases into one large tumour conglomerate. In the definition of the N classification, the perinodal compo-

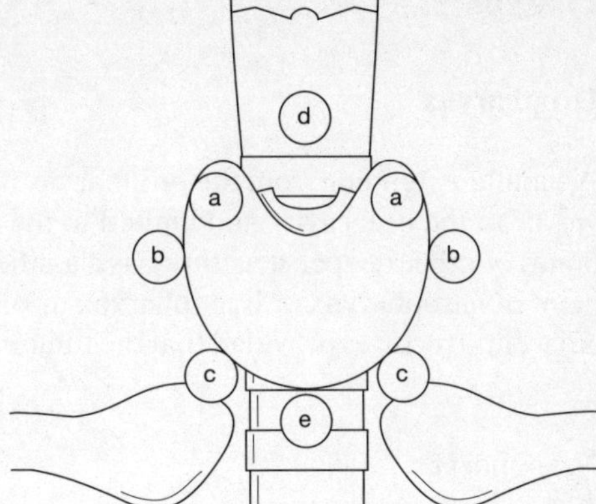

Fig. 9. Subdivision of prelaryngeal and paratracheal (anterior cervical) lymph nodes (group 8)

nent should be included in the size for isolated lymph node metastases; for conglomerates, the overall size of the conglomerate should be considered and not only the size of the individual lymph nodes.

Lip

Tumours that affect the vermilion surface as well as the skin are assigned to tumours of the lips when 50% or more of the tumour is within the vermilion surface.

The vermilion surface is demarcated from the mucosal surface by the line of contact of the opposing lips.

Oral Cavity

1. T4 definitions:
   a) The deep (extrinsic) muscle of the tongue includes musculi hyo-, stylo-, genio- and palatoglossus. Invasion indicates T4.
   b) The intrinsic muscle of the tongue includes musculi longitudinalis superior and inferior, transversus linguae and verticalis linguae. Invasion of the intrinsic muscle alone is not classified T4.
   c) Invasion up to cortical bone or erosion of the bone is not classified T4. There must be invasion through the cortical bone into the spongiosa.
2. A tumour extending from the oral cavity to the oropharynx and limited to the mucosa (without invasion of muscles, bones or other deeper structures) is classified only according to size. The involvement of oropharynx is not considered invasion of adjacent structures provided that the tumour is limited to the mucosa.

Pharynx

Oropharynx

A tumour extending from the oropharynx to the nasopharynx or to the hypopharynx or to the oral cavity and limited to the mucosa (without invasion of muscles, bones or other deeper structures) is classified only according to size. The involvement of nasopharynx or hypopharynx or oral cavity is not considered invasion of adjacent structures provided that the tumour is limited to the mucosa.

Nasopharynx

The term "postnasal space" corresponds to nasopharynx (C11). Invasion of vertebral bodies is classified T4.

Hypopharynx

1. The term "laryngopharynx" corresponds to hypopharynx (C13).
2. The hypopharyngeal surface of the aryepiglottic fold (C13.1) belongs to the hypopharynx, while the laryngeal aspect of the aryepiglottic fold (C32.1) is part of the supraglottis.
3. The uncommon tumours limited to one subsite but with fixation of hemilarynx should be classified as T3.
4. Fixation of hemilarynx is diagnosed endoscopically by immobility of the arytenoid.
5. Invasion of adjacent structures (T4) includes (see also p. 21):
   - Invasion of the thyroid or cricoid cartilage (involvement of perichondrium only is not invasion of the cartilage)
   - Invasion of the soft tissues of the neck
   - Invasion of vertebral bodies
6. Involvement of the arytenoid cartilage is classified as T3, not T4.

Larynx

Anatomical Definitions

Superior and Inferior Boundaries of the Glottis

According to the *AJCC Manual,* the inferior boundary of the supraglottis is the horizontal plane passing through the apex of the ventricle. However, the apex of the ventricle is an anatomically variable structure and is difficult to identify during endoscopy. Furthermore, Kleinsasser (1987, 1992) emphasized embryological and functional reasons for the following definition of the boundary between supraglottis and glottis:

> A plane running horizontally through the opening of the ventricle, posteriorly over the vocal process of the arytenoid cartilage and then rising between the cuneiform and the corniculate cartilage to end over the upper edge of the posterior commissure.

According to the *AJCC Manual,* the lower boundary of the glottis is the horizontal plane 1 cm below the apex of ventricle.

The designation "apex of ventricle" (AJCC 1992) and "the opening of the ventricle" (Kleinsasser 1987, 1992) are not mentioned in the anatomical international nomenclature; they correspond to the laryngeal saccule (sacculus larnygis, appendix ventriculi laryngis). To this definition the variability of the so-called apex and the difficulty of clinical endoscopic assessment have been opposed, and so the following definition is recommended (Steiner and Ambrosch 1993; see also Ogura and Mallen 1963; Alberti and Boyce 1976) (Fig. 10):

> The inferior boundary of the glottis is a horizontal plane 1 cm inferior to the level of the upper surface of the vocal cords, which divides supraglottis and glottis (Fig. 12).

It should be emphasized that Fleischer (1977), Glanz (1984) and Kleinsasser (1992) recommend that the differentiation between glottis and subglottis be dropped. There are embryological, clinical, histological and oncological reasons for combining glottis and subglottis carcinomas and classifying them according to a uniform schema (see extensive discussions by Kleinsasser 1992).

Subdivision of the Epiglottis

The epiglottis is divided by a plane passing the middle of the epiglottis (half-way between the free margin and the lower edge) (Kleinsasser and Glanz 1992). Steiner and Ambrosch (1993) propose dividing the epiglottis into the upper free part and the lower part which corresponds to the preepiglottic space. A horizontal plane between the bilateral pharyngoepiglottic fold represents the boundary. This plane may be recognized by endoscopy or radiologic imaging.

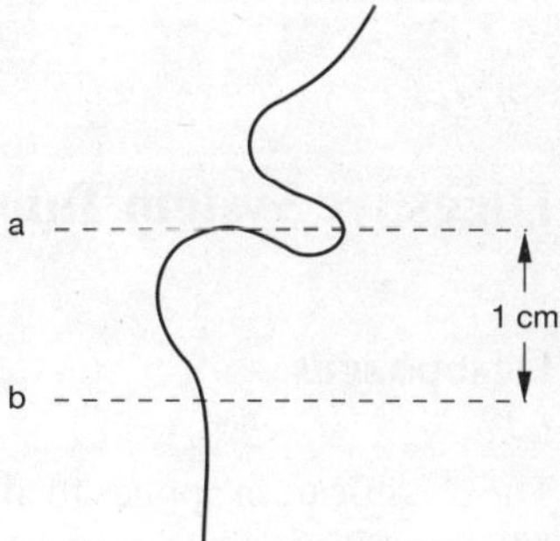

Fig. 10. Inferior boundary of the supraglottis (*a*) and inferior boundary of the glottis (*b*). (From Steiner and Ambrosch 1993)

Pathological Criteria of Impaired Vocal Cord Mobility or Vocal Cord Fixation

For pathological classification, impaired vocal cord mobility or fixation correspond to histological depth of invasion of more than 5 mm (Glanz 1984; Kleinsasser and Glanz 1992; Steiner and Ambrosch 1993; see also 113).

Associated Carcinoma in situ

1. In invasive carcinoma, the classification according to horizontal spread considers only the invasive component.
2. To indicate the presence of associated carcinoma in situ (adjacent or separated) the suffix "(is)" may be added to the respective T category of the invasive carcinoma, e. g. T2(is). The presence of an associated carcinoma in situ influences treatment of the invasive carcinoma and needs identification and separate analysis of such cases. An analogous procedure is already used for urinary bladder carcinoma.

Maxillary Sinus

Erosion of bone indicates that the tumour invades the cortex only; *invasion* of bone indicates that the spongiosa is involved.

Salivary Glands

Tumours arising in minor salivary glands localized in the mucous membrane of the upper aerodigestive tract are classified according to the rules for tumours of the oral cavity or pharynx.

Designation by histological type should be done to permit separation of squamous mucosal tumours from salivary gland tumours.

Digestive System Tumours

Oesophagus

The classification applies to all types of carcinoma, e. g. squamous cell carcinoma, adenocarcinoma in Barrett oesophagus and small cell carcinoma.

For the intrathoracic oesophagus, the regional lymph nodes are the mediastinal and the perigastric nodes excluding the coeliac nodes. These correspond to lymph node groups 1–7 according to the Japanese nomenclature (see p. 29).

Stomach

Anatomy

Gastric tumours located in the cardiac area may involve the distal oesophagus and primary oesophageal tumours may involve the cardiac area of the stomach. For differentiation between oesophageal and gastric carcinomas the following may be considered:

- If more than 50 % of the tumour involves the oesophagus, the tumour is classified as oesophageal; if less than 50 %, as gastric
- If the tumour is equally located above and below the oesophagogastric junction or is designated as being at the junction, squamous cell, small cell and undifferentiated carcinomas are classified as oesophageal, adenocarcinoma and signet ring cell carcinomas as gastric
- In the absence of Barrett oesophagus, an adenocarcinoma in both cardia and lower oesophagus is most likely to be gastric

Regional Lymph Nodes

The regional lymph nodes are:

- The perigastric nodes along the lesser curvature
    1 right cardiac
    3 lesser curvature
    5 suprapyloric
- The perigastric nodes along the greater curvature
    2 left cardiac
    4a greater curvature left
    4b greater curvature right
    6 infrapyloric
- The nodes located along the following arteries
    7 left gastric
    8 common hepatic
    9 coeliac
    10 splenic / at the splenic hilum
    11 splenic / along trunk

Note. The numerical order corresponds to the proposals of the Japanese Research Society for Gastric Cancer (1982)

In case of gastric stump carcinoma (following previous distal gastrectomy and localized at the anastomosis), lymph nodes in the mesentery of the intestinal loop used for anastomosis are classified as gastric regional nodes.

T Classification

Invasion of the transverse mesocolon is considered analogous to invasion of the gastrocolic ligament and is therefore classified T2 if the covering visceral peritoneum is not perforated (see TNM Classification 1992, Note 1, p. 46). The same applies to direct invasion of the greater omentum. Tumour nodules in the greater omentum which are separate from the primary tumour are classified as distant (peritoneal) metastasis (M1 PER).

Small Intestine

The very uncommon carcinoma in a Meckel diverticulum may be classified according to the classification for small intestine carcinoma, although supporting data are not available.

Intraluminal extension of an ileal carcinoma directly into the caecum (not by way of the serosa) does not affect the T classification, in particular does not qualify for T4.

Colon and Rectum

Anatomical Sites and Subsites

1. A tumour located at the border between two subsites is registered as a tumour of the subsite which is more involved.

   Example. Carcinoma with a longitudinal diameter of 6 cm, 2 cm in the caecum, 4 cm in the ascending colon, is classified as a carcinoma of the ascending colon.

   If two subsites are involved to the same extent, the lesion is classified as an overlapping lesion.

   Example. If the carcinoma involves 2 cm of the caecum and 2 cm of the ascending colon, the code C18.8 (overlapping lesion of the colon) is used.

2. The rectum is defined as the distal large intestine commencing opposite the sacral promontory and ending at the upper border of the anal canal. When measured from below with a rigid sigmoidoscope, it extends 16 cm from the anal verge. A tumour is classified as rectal if its lower margin lies less than 16 cm from the anal verge (Fielding et al. 1991). A tumour is considered rectal if any part is located at least partly within the supply of the superior rectal artery. Tumours are classified as rectosigmoid when differentiation between rectum and sigmoid according to the above rules is not possible.

Local Recurrence

A local recurrence after previous colon resection should be classified with the prefix "r" (for recurrence); the recurrent tumour is topographically assigned to the proximal segment of the anastomosis.

Regional Lymph Nodes

Lymph nodes along the course of a named vascular trunk are the nodes located along the following, and their involvement is classified N3:

- Ileocolic artery
- Right colic artery
- Middle colic artery
- Left colic artery
- Inferior mesenteric artery
- Superior rectal (superior haemorrhoidal) artery
- Internal iliac artery

Note. Nodes along the sigmoid arteries are considered pericolic nodes; their involvement is classified N1 or N2 (according to the number involved).

For each anatomical subsite the following are the specific named vascular trunks:

Appendix	ileocolic
Caecum	ileocolic and right colic
Ascending colon	ileocolic, right colic and middle colic
Hepatic flexure	middle colic and right colic
Transverse colon	right colic, middle colic, left colic and inferior mesenteric
Splenic flexure	middle colic, left colic and inferior mesenteric
Descending colon	middle colic, left colic and inferior mesenteric
Sigmoid colon } Rectosigmoid }	left colic, superior rectal (haemorrhoidal) and inferior mesenteric
Rectum	superior rectal (haemorrhoidal), inferior mesenteric and internal iliac

Metastasis in nodes along a named vascular trunk other than those listed is classified as distant metastasis, e. g. metastasis in a node along the middle colic artery in a case of rectal carcinoma is M1.

Perirectal nodes include the mesorectal (paraproctal), lateral sacral, presacral, sacral promotory (Gerota), middle rectal (haemorrhoidal) and inferior rectal (haemorrhoidal) nodes. Metastasis in the external iliac or common iliac nodes is classified as distant metastasis.

Involvement of "apical nodes" corresponds to involvement of the nodes along the course of the respective named vascular trunk (N3).

The pericolic nodes correspond to "epicolic" and "paracolic" nodes according to the division of Jamieson and Dobson (1909) ("epicolic", on the colon itself; "paracolic", along the marginal artery and between it and the colon). Jamieson and Dobson's "intermediate nodes" include nodes on the branches of the major colic vessels, now classified as pericolic, as well as nodes along the course of a named vascular trunk. The "principal glands" of Jamieson and Dobson include the nodes on the inferior mesenteric artery and on the superior mesenteric artery, the latter to be classified as nonregional.

T/pT Classification

1. For colon and rectum only, Tis/pTis (carcinoma in situ) includes cases with invasion of the lamina propria (including the muscularis mucosae but not of the submucosa), i. e. intramucosal, as well as intraepithelial carcinoma.
2. T3/pT3: The perirectal tissue includes the mesorectum (paraproctium).
3. A free perforation of a colorectal carcinoma into the peritoneal cavity is classified as T4.
4. *Intramural* direct extension from one subsite (segment) of the colon to an adjacent one is not considered in the T classification. The same applies to *intramural* direct extension from the rectum to the sigmoid colon and vice versa and from the rectum to the anal canal.
5. *Intramural* extension of a caecal carcinoma directly into the ileum (not by way of serosa) does not affect the T classification, in particular does not qualify for T4. In contrast, direct extension via serosa or via mesocolon is classified T4, e. g. extension of a sigmoid colon carcinoma to caecum.
6. Tumour cells in veins or lymphatics do not affect the pT classification. The L and V classifications can be used to record such spread.

   Example. Carcinoma with continuous local spread into the submucosa, tumour cells in a small vein within the muscularis propria – pT1.

N/pN Classification

A tumour nodule greater than 3 mm in diameter in the perirectal or pericolic adipose tissue without histological evidence of a residual node in the nodule is classified as regional perirectal/pericolic lymph node metastasis. However, a tumour nodule up to 3 mm in diameter is classified in the T category as discontinuous extension, i. e. T3.

Anal Canal

Rules for Classification

The classification applies to all types of carcinoma including those arising within an anorectal fistula as well as squamous cell (cloacogenic) carcinoma

T Classification

Direct invasion of rectal wall or perirectal skin or subcutaneous perianal tissue is not considered T4. The tumour is classified by size.

Liver

Rules for Classification

At present, the classification applies to carcinomas of intrahepatic bile ducts (cholangiocellular carcinoma) as well as hepatocellular carcinoma.

Regional Lymph Nodes

Hilar nodes include those at the hepatic pedicle and those along the inferior vena cava, proper hepatic artery and portal vein. The inferior phrenic lymph nodes are nonregional.

T/pT Classification

1. "Multiplicity" includes multiple nodules representing multiple, independent primary tumours as well as intrahepatic metastasis from a single primary hepatic carcinoma
2. "Vascular invasion" is diagnosed clinically by imaging procedures. In the pathological classification it includes gross as well as histological involvement of vessels.
3. T4: "major branches of the portal or hepatic veins" are the right and left branches of the portal vein and the corresponding veins (not segmental or subsegmental branches). Involvement of the right, left and (not always existent) intermediate branches of the hepatic artery is also classified T4.
4. Invasion of adjacent organs is not mentioned in the T classification. It is recommended to classify tumours with direct invasion of adjacent organs other than the gallbladder as T4. Perforation of the visceral peritoneum should be classified T4, too.
5. Direct invasion of gallbladder is disregarded because it influences neither treatment nor prognosis.

Gallbladder

Carcinoma of the cystic duct is classified as a tumour of the extrahepatic bile ducts. For a definition of hilar nodes see Liver (above).

Extrahepatic Bile Ducts

The extrahepatic bile ducts include:

- Left and right hepatic ducts (tumours arising here are often referred to as hilar carcinomas of the liver)

– Common hepatic duct
– Cystic duct
– Common bile duct (choledochus)

This classification does not apply to carcinomas of the ampulla of Vater.
For the definition of hilar nodes, see p. 33.
Direct invasion of the portal vein or the hepatic artery is classified T3.

A question has been raised (Murakata 1993) regarding the presence of a muscle layer in the extrahepatic bile ducts in reference to the T definitions. The muscle layer in this area is only prominent in the distal part of the common duct. Proximally instead of a distinct muscle layer there is a zone of dense connective tissue with some muscle fibers. Invasion of this fibromuscular zone corresponds to T1b, while invasion of the loose connective tissue beyond this zone is classified T2.

Ampulla of Vater

The ampulla opens into the duodenum through a small mucosal elevation, the duodenal papilla or papilla of Vater. Tumours of the ampulla of Vater include tumours arising in the ampulla, tumours arising on the papilla and tumours arising at the junction of the mucosa of the ampulla with that of the papilla.

Pancreas

T Classification

T2   Peripancreatic tissues include the surrounding retroperitoneal fat (retroperitoneal soft tissue or retroperitoneal space), including the mesentery (mesenteric fat), mesocolon, greater and lesser omentum and peritoneum.
Direct invasion to bile ducts and duodenum includes involvement of the ampulla of Vater.

T3   Adjacent large vessels are the portal vein, the coeliac artery and the superior mesenteric and common hepatic arteries and veins (not the splenic vessels).

Lung Tumours

T Classification (Mountain et al. 1992)

1. Invasion of phrenic nerve is classified as T3.
2. Vocal cord paralysis (resulting from invasion of the recurrent branch of the vagus nerve), superior vena caval obstruction or compression of the trachea or oesophagus is classified as T4.

3. T4: the "great vessels" are
   - Aorta
   - Superior vena cava
   - Inferior vena cava
   - Main pulmonary artery (pulmonary trunk)
   - Intrapericardial portions of the right and left pulmonary artery
   - Intrapericardial portions of the superior and inferior right and left pulmonary veins

Invasion of more distal branches does not qualify for classification as T4.

4. Direct extension to parietal pericardium is classified T3 and to visceral pericardium, T4.
5. Tumour foci in the ipsilateral parietal and visceral pleura that are discontinuous from direct pleural invasion by the primary tumour are classified T4.
6. Pericardial effusion is classified the same as pleural effusion.
7. In case of clinically or grossly multiple tumour foci in the ipsilateral lung, i. e. satellite nodule(s) or other nodule(s) in the same lobe or in another ipsilateral lobe(s), the primary tumour should be "up-staged" according to the following rules:
   a) For satellite lesion(s) or additional tumour nodule(s) in the same lobe, T1 should be up-staged to T2, T2 to T3 and T3 to T4
   b) Primary tumour with additional nodule(s) in another ipsilateral lobe, regardless of site or location of the primary, should be classified as T4.

M Classification

1. Discontinuous tumour lesions outside the parietal pleura in the chest wall or in the diaphragm are classified M1 (Mountain et al. 1992).
2. All primary and metastatic disease in one hemithorax, except discontinuous lesions in the chest wall and diaphragm, should be reflected in the T and N classifications. The M classification is reserved for more distant sites of disease. Therefore, the definitions of M0 and M1 should read:

M0   No distant metastasis outside the ipsilateral hemithorax

M1   Distant metastasis outside the ipsilateral hemithorax (metastasis to ipsi- and/or contralateral supraclavicular and scalene lymph nodes are not considered as distant metastasis and classified N3)

Small Cell Carcinoma

The TNM classification and stage grouping should be generally applied to small cell carcinoma. TNM is of significance for prognosis of small cell carcinoma, too (Mountain 1988), and has the advantage of providing a uniform detailed classification of tumour spread. The former categories "limited" and "extensive" for small cell carcinoma have been inconsistently defined and used.

The category "limited disease" as used in the Veterans Administration Lung Cancer Study Group system for classification of small cell carcinoma (Hyde et al.

1965) corresponds to stages I to III A and "extensive disease" to stages III B ("extensive disease I") and IV ("extensive disease II").

Multiple Synchronous Primary Tumours

If histologically confirmed synchronous multiple primary lung cancers are present, classification should follow the general rule no. 5 of the TNM Classification 1992 (see p. 3). If indeterminate bilateral tumours are present, one tumour should be designated as the primary tumour and the contralateral tumour as distant metastasis.

Bone Tumours

Skip metastasis in the same bone as the primary is not considered in the TNM classification. Metastasis in another bone is classified as distant metastasis.

Soft Tissue Tumours

A TNM classification and stage grouping of Kaposi sarcoma are not provided. The prognosis of Kaposi sarcoma associated with AIDS is determined by AIDS.

Skin Tumours

Carcinoma of Skin

1. The classification applies to any type of skin carcinoma: squamous cell, basal cell, skin appendages, Merkel cell.
2. The classification does not apply to carcinomas of the eyelid, vulva and penis. They have separate classifications.
3. In carcinoma of the perianal skin (anal margin), direct invasion of the mucosa or submucosa of the anal canal does not affect the T/pT classification. The tumour is classified by size.
4. Metastatic involvement of iliac and other pelvic, abdominal or intrathoracic lymph nodes is classified as M1

Malignant Melanoma of Skin

1. The classification applies to malignant melanoma of skin of all sites, including eyelid, vulva, penis and scrotum. It does not apply to melanomas arising in mucous membranes (oral cavity, nasopharynx, vagina, urethra, anal canal) or to melanomas of the conjunctiva and uvea. The last two sites have separate classifications. There is no classification for melanoma of the oral cavity, nasopharynx or other visceral sites.
2. The pT classification of malignant melanoma considers three histological criteria:
   - Maximum tumour thickness (Breslow) according to the largest vertical diameter of the tumour in millimetres.
   Maximum thickness of the tumour is measured with an ocular micrometer after embedding in paraffin at right angles to the adjacent normal skin. The upper reference point is the top of the granular cell layer of the epidermis of the overlying skin or the base of the ulcer if the tumour is ulcerated. The lower reference point is usually the deepest point of invasion. It may be the invading edge of a single tumour mass or an isolated cell or group of cells deep to the main mass. Melanoma cells within the epithelium of structures such as hair follicles and sebaceous glands of the skin are not taken into consideration.
   - Clark levels.
   - Absence or presence of satellites within 2 cm of the primary tumour. "Satellites" include tumour nests and nodules not only in the dermis but also in the subcutaneous tissue.

   The definitive pT category is based on these three criteria. In case of discrepancy between tumour thickness and level, the pT category is based on the less favourable finding (Fig. 11).
3. In-transit metastases without regional lymph node metastasis or with regional lymph node metastasis 3 cm or less in greatest dimension are classified N2b.

Thickness (mm) / Clark levels	II	III	IV	V
-0.75	pT1			
> 0.75 to 1.50		pT2		
> 0.75 to 3.00			pT3a	
> 3.00 to 4.00		pT3b		
> 4.00				pT4a
Satellites		pT4b		

Fig. 11. pT classification of malignant melanoma. (From TNM Atlas 1992)

Breast Tumours

Rules for Classification

1. The classification applies to carcinomas of the male as well as of the female breast.
2. The rules for multiple simultaneous primary cancers in one breast (see p. 3) do not apply to a single grossly detected tumour associated with multiple separate *microscopic* foci (satellites).

Regional Lymph Nodes

Intramammary lymph nodes are coded as axillary lymph nodes level I.

T Classification

1. The clinical estimation of tumour size by physical examination and mammography frequently give different results (Fornage et al. 1987; Pain et al. 1992). Accuracy can be improved by using the following formula:

    Size for classification $= 0.5 \times$ physical examination size
    $+ 0.5 \times$ mammographic size (Pain et al. 1992).
2. Only clinically/grossly detected satellite skin nodules are classified T4b (histologically detected foci are not considered).
3. Dimpling of the skin, nipple retraction, nipple involvement or other skin changes, except those in T4b and T4d, may occur in T1, T2 or T3 without affecting the classification. This also applies to microscopic invasion of the skin (dermis) without changes of T4b or T4d.
4. On mastectomy specimens oedema of the skin (T4b) may be inapparent at the time of pathological examination. Therefore, the surgeon should inform the pathologist of such a clinical finding to guarantee its consideration and to prevent pathological understaging.

N/pN Classification

The N classification is done by the clinical and imaging methods usually applied for examination of the axilla. At the present time, special efforts are not required for evaluation of internal mammary lymph nodes (N3).

pN1 (movable nodes) and pN2 (nodes that are fixed to one another or to other structures) are differentiated by macroscopic findings of the pathologist during dissection of the axillary specimen.

Gynaecological Tumours

Vulva

The classification for vulva was changed in 1989 by FIGO. It was adopted by the UICC and AJCC and published in the Corrected Reprint of the TNM Atlas (1990) and the TNM Classification, Revision 1992.

Invasion of the rectal wall or bladder wall (not mucosa) is classified as T3. Mucosal involvement is T4.

Vagina

"Frozen pelvis" is a clinical term which means that tumour extends to the pelvic wall(s). It is classified as T3.

Invasion of the rectal wall or bladder wall (not mucosa) is classified as T2. Mucosal involvement is T4.

Cervix Uteri

Regional Lymph Nodes

The designations "internal iliac" and "hypogastric" are synonyms.

T Classification

T1a1 or FIGO IA1 (minimal stromal invasion) applies to lesions with minute foci of invasion visible only microscopically.

T1a2 or FIGO IA2 is used for lesions macroscopically measurable on the slide (even if dots need to be placed on the slide prior to assessment). Venous or lymphatic invasion does not alter classification (FIGO 1991).

The presence of tumour cells in lymphatics of the parametrium does not qualify for T2b. T2b is used only for grossly evident continuous invasion beyond the myometrium.

"Frozen pelvis" is a clinical term which means that tumour extends to the pelvic wall(s), i. e. T3b.

Invasion of the rectal wall or bladder wall (not mucosa) is classified as T3a. Mucosal involvement is T4.

Corpus Uteri

The classification for corpus uteri was changed in 1989 by FIGO. It was adopted by the UICC and AJCC and published in the 1990 Revision of the TNM Atlas and the TNM Classification, Revision 1992.

Regional Lymph Nodes

The designations "internal iliac" and "hypogastric" are synonyms.

T Classification

T3a or FIGO IIIA includes discontinuous involvement of adnexae or serosa within the pelvis.

Invasion of the rectal wall or bladder wall (not mucosa) is classified as T3b. Mucosal involvement is T4.

"Frozen pelvis" is a clinical term which means that tumour extends to the pelvic wall(s), i. e. T3b.

There may be a small number of patients with T1 corpus carcinoma who will be treated primarily with radiation therapy. For these cases FIGO recommends clinical classification according to the former FIGO schedule (IA, uterine cavity 8 cm or less in length; IB, uterine cavity more than 8 cm in length), but the use of this staging system must be stated.

Ovary

The TNM classification and FIGO staging are also applicable to carcinomas designated "borderline" or "of low malignant potential".

Regional Lymph Nodes

The designations "internal iliac" and "hypogastric" are synonyms.

T Classification

T1c   Rupture of the capsule includes spontaneous rupture as well as rupture caused by the surgeon.

T2/3   The "pelvis" includes the true or minor or small as well as the false major or large or false pelvis.

T3   Peritoneal metastasis outside the pelvis includes involvement of the omentum.

Microscopic confirmation of a single peritoneal metastasis outside the pelvis, irrespective of the size of the metastasis, is required for T3. For the subdivision size alone is relevant. Therefore, T3c is appropriate based on the macroscopic assessment by the surgeon even if microscopic confirmation was of a smaller metastasis only.

M Classification

In ovary, peritoneal metastasis is not considered distant metastasis; it is classified as T3.

Urological Tumours

Penis

Erythroplasia of Queyrat is classified as carcinoma in situ (Tis).

Prostate

T Classification

When a tumour is an incidental finding in transurethral resection (TUR) and after the first TUR a repeated TUR (re-TUR) is performed within 2 months as part of the definitive primary treatment (without following radical prostatectomy), the subdivision into T1a and T1b should be based on the findings of both TURs.

Examples
1. First TUR: <5% of tissue resected involved by carcinoma. Re-TUR with the same amount of tissue: 10% of tissue involved. Classify T1b.
2. First TUR: 10% of tissue resected involved by carcinoma. Re-TUR including a threefold amount of tissue: no further tumour found. Classify T1a.

If a TUR has incidental carcinoma (T1a or T1b) and a subsequent radical prostatectomy specimen has no residual tumour, the classification is pT1.

The pathological classification of tumours in radical prostatectomy specimens confined within the prostate depends on the clinical information available to the pathologist: if the pathologist has knowledge of the negative palpation and imaging findings (incidental carcinoma) the classification is pT1 (a or b), otherwise the tumour is classified pT2.

Involvement of the prostatic urethra is not considered in the T classification.

"Frozen pelvis" is a clinical term which means that tumour extends to the pelvic wall(s) and is fixed. It is classified as T4.

Histopathological Grading

The Gleason score and Gleason pattern (Gleason and VACURG 1977) correspond to the grading recommended here as follows:

Gleason score	Gleason pattern	UICC/AJCC histopathological grade
2–4	1, 2	1
5–7	3	2
8–10	4, 5	3–4

Testis

1. Synchronous bilateral tumours should be staged separately as independent primary tumours.
2. pT2: Invasion beyond the tunica albuginea includes invasion of any of the following: cremaster muscle, cremaster fascia, testicular portion of the internal or external spermatic fascia. Invasion beyond these structures into the subcutis or cutis of the scrotum is classified as pT4.
3. pT3: Invasion of the spermatic cord refers to direct extension. Tumour cells in vessels of the spermatic cord are not considered in the T classification. The L and V classifications can be used to record invasion of vessels in the spermatic cord.

Kidney

Gerota fascia (renal fascia) includes the pre- and retrorenal fascia. Invasion of the peritoneum is invasion beyond the Gerota fascia (prerenal fascia) and is classified as T4.

Renal Pelvis and Ureter

1. Direct extension into the urinary bladder in the region of the ostium is classified by the depth of greatest invasion in any of the involved organs.
2. In tumours of the ureter, adjacent organs include parietal peritoneum.

3. The prognosis of T3 in ureter is worse than in renal pelvis and corresponds approximately to T4 renal pelvis tumours. Therefore, separate analysis of ureter and renal pelvis carcinoma is recommended (Guinan et al. 1992).
4. For classification of multiple synchronous primary tumours renal pelvis and ureter are considered a single organ. Therefore, in case of synchronous tumours in the renal pelvis and the ureter, the tumour with the highest T category should be classified and the multiplicity or the number of tumours should be indicated in parentheses, e. g. T2(m) or T3(2). In contrast, in case of synchronous tumours in the renal pelvis and the urinary bladder, both tumours should be classified independently.

Urinary Bladder

1. If the pathology specimen does not contain muscle, the category T1 is applicable (see TNM Classification 1992, general rule no. 4). However, the pathology report should state the absence of muscle to allow the clinician to consider repeating the biopsy.
2. In case of transurethral resection, differentiation between T2 and T3a is possible only if the surgeon submits the material separated into a superficial (inner) and deep (outer) portion and histological examination is performed separately. Otherwise, the case is classified as T2 (according to TNM Classification 1992, general rule no. 4).
3. Direct invasion of the distal ureter is classified by the depth of greatest invasion in any of the involved organs.
4. Uncommonly, carcinomas of the bladder neck show an associated in situ component extending into the prostatic ducts and sometimes into the prostatic glands without any invasion in the prostate. Such cases are classified according to the depth of bladder wall invasion. The extension of the associated in situ component into the prostate does not qualify for classification as T4. It may be indicated by the suffix "(is)", e. g. T2(is).
5. Involvement of prostatic urethra is included in prostatic involvement and is therefore classified as T4.
6. Direct invasion of the large or small intestine should be classified as T4. The same applies to invasion through the peritoneum covering the bladder.

Recurrent Carcinoma after Cystectomy and Ureterosigmoidostomy

A recurrent transitional carcinoma in the region of a ureterosigmoidostomy may invade only the subepithelial connective tissue of the ureter and the adjacent mucosa and submucosa of the sigmoid colon. In this case the invasion of the colon should not be considered as invasion of an adjacent organ. For the T classification the rules for ureter and colon should be applied, i. e. rT1 is the correct classification.

Urethra

In urethral diverticular carcinoma a differentiation between T2 and T3 is not possible (Clayton et al. 1992). In this case the T category "T2–3" is used.

Ophthalmic Tumours

Carcinoma of Eyelid

The eyelids are covered externally by epidermis (anterior surface of the eyelid) and internally by conjunctiva (posterior surface). This classification applies only to the carcinomas of the anterior surface of the eyelid and the eyelid margin. Carcinomas of the posterior surface of the eyelid are considered under tumours of the conjunctiva.

Malignant Melanoma of Eyelid

This classification applies only to malignant melanoma of the anterior surface of the eyelid. Melanoma of the posterior surface of the eyelid is considered under melanoma of the conjunctiva.

Carcinoma of Conjunctiva

This classification applies to carcinoma of the palpebral and bulbar conjunctiva and the conjunctival fornix.

Malignant Melanoma of Conjunctiva

This classification applies to malignant melanoma of the palpebral and bulbar conjunctiva and the conjunctival fornix.

Involvement of eyelid is defined as invasion beyond the tarsal plate into the anterior part of the eyelid.

Brain Tumours

The classification applies to the following brain tumours (Zülch 1979):

1. Astrocytomas
2. Oligodendrogliomas
3. Ependymal and choroid plexus tumours
4. Glioblastoma
5. Medulloblastoma
6. Meningioma, malignant
7. Neurilemmoma (neurinoma, schwannoma), malignant
8. Haemangioblastoma
9. Neurosarcoma
10. Other sarcomas

Tumours should be separated by histological type for valid comparisons.

Invasion of dura, cranial nerves, spinal cord, bones and adjacent organs, e.g. nasopharynx, paranasal sinus, is classified as T4.

Lymph node metastases are not observed because there are no lymphatic structures draining the brain. Seeding into the subarachnoid space or into ventricles is classified as distant metastasis.

Hodgkin Disease and Non-Hodgkin Lymphomas

1. Single lymph node regions are:
   - Lymph nodes of head, face and neck
   - Intrathoracic lymph nodes
   - Intra-abdominal lymph nodes
   - Lymph nodes of axilla or arm
   - Lymph nodes of inguinal region or leg
   - Pelvic lymph nodes

Examples

Involvement	Classification
Parotid and jugular	Single node region
Jugular and tracheal	Two regions, same side of diaphragm
Tracheal, hilar, para-aortic abdominal	Two regions, both sides of diaphragm

2. Direct spread of a lymphoma into adjacent tissues or organs does not influence classification.

   Examples
   - Lymphoma of a cervical lymph node with pericapsular extension into adjacent muscle – stage I

- Gastric lymphoma with direct spread to pancreas and involvement of perigastric lymph nodes – stage II_E
- Lymphoma involving the ascending colon, caecum and ileocaecal valve with direct extension to the terminal ileum – stage I_E

3. Involvement of two or more segments of the gastrointestinal tract, isolated and not in continuity, is classified as stage IV (disseminated involvement of one or more extralymphatic organs).

   Example. Involvement of stomach and of ileum – stage IV.

4. For classification of extranodal lymphomas, involvement of both organs of a paired site is considered as involvement of a single organ.

   Example. Extranodal lymphoma involving both lungs is classified stage I_E.

5. Multifocal involvement of a single extralymphatic organ is classified stage I_E and not stage IV.

6. Primary Extranodal Lymphomas, Stage II_E: The definitions of regional lymph nodes given for the individual tumour sites apply to extranodal lymphomas, too, e. g. for primary gastric lymphomas the regional lymph nodes are the perigastric nodes along the lesser and greater curvatures and the nodes located along the left gastric, common hepatic, splenic and coeliac arteries.

   For further explanatory notes see p. 45.

Paediatric Tumours

Soft Tissue Sarcomas – Paediatric

1. The classification is used for patients below the age of 15 years. While the classification of soft tissue sarcomas in adults does not apply to sarcomas arising from parenchymatous organs or hollow viscera, the classification of paediatric sarcomas does apply to such sarcomas, e. g. sarcomas of the vagina, urinary bladder or extrahepatic bile ducts.
2. In case of tumours in the midline or in the other boundary zones, multidirectional lymph drainage occurs. For the definition of regional lymph nodes in this situation, see the rules described in detail under the classification of skin tumours (TNM Classification 1992, p. 94). For a sarcoma of the diaphragm, the mediastinal as well as the abdominal lymph nodes are regional.

References

Alberti PW, Boyce DB (eds) (1976) Workshops from the centennial conference on laryngeal cancer. Appleton Century Crofts, New York

Clayton M, Siami F, Guinan P (1992) Urethral diverticular carcinoma. Cancer 70: 665–670

Dralle H (1992) Personal communication

Fielding LP, Arsenault PA, Chapuis PH, Dent O, Gatright B, Hardcastle JD, Hermanek P, Jass JR, Newland RC (1991) Clinicopathological staging for colorectal cancer: an International Documentation System (IDS) and an International Comprehensive Anatomical Terminology (ICAT). J Gastroenterol Hepatol 6: 325–344

FIGO (1991) Annual report on the results of treatment in gynecological cancer, vol 21. Elsevier, Amsterdam

Fleischer I (1977) Morphologische Untersuchungen an subglottischen Kehlkopfcarcinomen. Inaugural dissertation, University Marburg, FRG

Fornage BD, Tonbas O, Morel M (1987) Clinical, mammographic, and sonographic determination of preoperative breast cancer size. Cancer 60: 765–771

Glanz HK (1984) Carcinoma of the larynx. Growth, p-classification and grading of squamous cell carcinoma of the vocal cords. Adv Oto-Rhino-Laryngol 32: 1–123

Gleason DF, Veterans Administration Cooperative Urological Research Group (VACURG) (1977) Histologic grading and clinical staging of prostatic carcinoma. In: Tannenbaum M (Ed) Urologic pathology: the prostate. Lea and Febiger, Philadelphia

Guinan P, Volgelzang NJ, Randazzo R, Fremgen A, Chmiel J, Sylvester J, Sener S (1992) Renal pelvic transitional cell carcinoma. The role of the kidney in tumor-node-metastasis staging. Cancer 69: 1773–1775

Hyde L, Yee J, Wilson R, Patno ME (1965) Cell type and the natural history of lung cancer. JAMA 193: 52–54

Jamieson JK, Dobson JF (1909) The lymphatics of the colon. Proc R Soc Med 2: 149–152

Japanese Research Society for Gastric Cancer (1982) General rules for the gastric cancer study in surgery and pathology. Jap J Surg 11: 127–145

Kleinsasser O (1987) Tumoren des Larynx und des Hypopharynx. Thieme, Stuttgart

Kleinsasser O (1992) Revision of classification of laryngeal cancer, is it long overdue? (Proposals for an improved TN-classification) J Laryngol Otol 106: 197–204

Kleinsasser O, Glanz H (1992) Personal communication

Mountain CF (1988) Prognostic implications of the international staging system for lung. Semin Oncol 15: 236–245

Mountain CF, Libshitz HI, Hermes KE (1992) Lung cancer. A handbook for staging and imaging. Ch P Young Comp, Houston

Murakata LA (1993) Personal communication

Ogura JH, Powers WE, Holtz S, Mc Gavran MH, Ellis B, Voorhees R (1960) Laryngograms; their value in the diagnosis and treatment of laryngeal lesions. Laryngoscope 70: 780–809

Pain JA, Ebbs SR, Hern RPA, Lowe S, Bradbeer JW (1992) Assessment of breast cancer size: a comparison of methods. Eur J Surg Oncol 18: 44–48

Robbins KT, Medina JE, Wolfe GT, Levine PA, Sessions RB, Pruet CW (1991) Standardizing neck dissection terminology. Official report of the Academy's Committee for Head and Neck Surgery and Oncology. Arch Otolaryngol Head Neck Surg 117: 601–605

Steiner W, Ambrosch P (1993) A proposal for a modified T classification of head and neck tumors. Otorhinolaryngologica nova (in press)

Watanabe H, Jass JR, Sobin LH (1990) Histological typing of oesophageal and gastric tumours. 2nd edn. Springer, Berlin Heidelberg New York (WHO international histological classification of tumours)

Zeng Z, Cohen AM, Hajdu S, Sternberg SS, Sigurdson ER, Enker W (1992) Serosal cytologic study to determine free mesothelial penetration by intraperitoneal colon cancer. Cancer 70: 737–740

Zülch KJ (1979) Histological typing of tumours of the central nervous system. WHO, Geneva (WHO international histological classification of tumours)

Site-Specific Recommendations
for pT and pN

Introduction

This chapter is an expansion to the following general rules of the TNM system
(TNM Classification 1992, pp. 5, 6):

> 2 b. Pathological assessment of the primary tumour (pT) entails a resection of
> the primary tumour or biopsy adequate to evaluate the highest pT category.
> The pathological assessment of the regional lymph nodes (pN) entails re-
> moval of nodes adequate to validate the absence of regional lymph node
> metastasis (pNO) and sufficient to evaluate the highest pN category.
> 4. If there is doubt concerning the correct T, N or M category to which a partic-
> ular case should be allotted, then the lower (i. e. less advanced) category
> should be chosen.

In the TNM Classification (1992) these general rules have been specified for breast
cancer only. Analogous definitions for the other tumour sites are given below.

The classification pN0 requires a regional lymphadenectomy and the histological examination of the specimen. The number of lymph nodes ordinarily included in the respective lymphadenectomy specimens is stated below. These numbers are considered adequate for staging. If the examined lymph nodes are
negative, but the number ordinarily resected is not met, classify as pNO. The number of nodes examined and the number involved by tumour should be recorded in
the pathology report (Qizilbash 1982; Remmele 1984; Honthoff 1989; Hermanek
et al. 1989, Rosai 1989; Fielding et al. 1991). This information may also be added in
parentheses, e. g. pN0 (0/11) or pN 1 (4/12).

In many tumour sites, the number of involved regional lymph nodes indicates
differences in prognosis. For details see pp. 101 ff. A correlation exists between the
number of examined lymph nodes and the pN classification. With increasing number of examined lymph nodes a higher frequency of lymph node-positive cases is
found and – in tumour sites where more than one positive pN category is provided
– a greater proportion of higher pN categories can be observed. Examples are
shown for stomach, colorectum and malignant melanoma in Appendices 1–3 on
pp. 68–70. Therefore, the number of examined lymph nodes reflects the reliability
of pN classification.

Head and Neck Tumours

pT – Primary Tumour

Site	pT 3 or less Recommendation for all sites	pT 4 microscopic confirmation of:
Lip	Pathological examination of the primary carcinoma with *no gross tumour* at the margins of resection (with or without microscopic involvement)	Invasion of spongious bone, tongue or skin of neck
Oral Cavity		Invasion of spongious bone, deep (extrinsic) muscle of tongue, maxillary sinus or skin
Oropharynx		Invasion of spongious bone, soft tissue of neck or deep (extrinsic) muscle of tongue
Nasopharynx		Invasion of skull or cranial nerve
Hypopharynx		Invasion of cartilage or soft tissues of neck
Larynx		Invasion of tissue beyond the larynx, e. g. on the outer side of thyroid or cricoid cartilage or soft tissues of neck
Maxillary Sinus		Invasion of the orbital content and/or of the following: cribriform plate, posterior ethmoid or sphenoid sinuses, nasopharyx, soft palate, pterygomaxillary or temporal fossae, base of skull
Salivary Glands		As for pT3
Thyroid Gland		Invasion of tissue beyond the thyroid capsule

pN – Regional Lymph Nodes

Site	Recommendations

All Sites Except Thyroid Gland

pN0, pN1
Histological examination of a selective neck dissection specimen which will ordinarily include 6 or more lymph nodes *or* Histological examination of a radical or modified radical neck dissection specimen which will ordinarily include 10 or more lymph nodes

pN2
Microscopic confirmation of a regional lymph node metastasis more than 3 cm but not more than 6 cm in greatest dimension *or* Microscopic confirmation of at least two regional lymph node metastases, none more than 6 cm in greatest dimension

pN3
Microscopic confirmation of a regional lymph node metastasis more than 6 cm in greatest dimension

Notes. 1. Terminology of neck dissection (Robbins et al. 1991): A radical neck dissection includes the removal of all ipsilateral cervical lymph node groups, i.e. lymph nodes from levels I through V (see p. 24), and removal of the spinal accessory nerve, internal jugular vein and sternocleidomastoid muscle.

In a modified radical neck dissection the same lymph nodes are removed as in a radical neck dissection; however, one or more nonlymphatic structures are preserved.

A selective neck dissection is a neck dissection with preservation of one or more lymph node groups routinely removed in radical neck dissection.

The most often performed types of selective neck dissections are: (a) supraomohyoid dissection; levels I–III; (b) posterolateral neck dissection, levels II–V and the retroauricular and occipital (suboccipital) nodes; (c) lateral neck dissection, levels II–IV; (d) anterior compartment neck dissection, level VI.

2. If the size of a *biopsied* lymph node is not indicated by the submitting surgeon, classify pN1 if the positive biopsy is from one node; and pN2 if positive biopsies are from two or more lymph nodes.

Thyroid Gland

pNO
Histological examination of a selective neck dissection specimen which will ordinarily include 6 or more lymph nodes

pN1a
As for pN0, or positive biopsy from an ipsilateral cervical lymph node

pN1b
Microscopic confirmation of a midline or contralateral cervical or mediastinal lymph node metastasis

Digestive System Tumours

pT – Primary Tumour

Site	Recommendations
Oesophagus	**pT3 or less** Pathological examination of the primary carcinoma with *no gross tumour* at the deep (radial, lateral), proximal and distal margins of the resection (with or without microscopic involvement) **pT4** Microscopic confirmation of invasion of adjacent structures
Stomach	**pT3 or less** Pathological examination of the primary carcinoma removed by total or partial gastrectomy with *no gross tumour* at the deep (radial, lateral), proximal and distal margins of resection (with or without microscopic involvement) *or* Pathological examination of the primary carcinoma removed by endoscopic polypectomy or local excision with histologically tumour-free margins of resection **pT4** Microscopic confirmation of invasion of adjacent structures such as spleen, transverse colon, liver, diaphragm, pancreas, abdominal wall, adrenal gland, kidney, small intestine and/or retroperitoneum
Small Intestine	**pT3 or less** Pathological examination of the primary carcinoma removed by short segment (limited) or radical resection with *no gross tumour* at the deep (radial, lateral), proximal and distal margins of resection (with or without microscopic involvement) *or* Pathological examination of the primary carcinoma removed by endoscopic polypectomy or local excision with histologically tumour-free margins of resection **pT4** Pathological confirmation[1] of perforation of the visceral peritoneum *or* Microscopic confirmation of invasion of other organs or structures (including other loops of small intestine, mesentery or retroperi-

toneum more than 2 cm and abdominal wall via serosa; for duodenum only, invasion of pancreas)

Colon and Rectum

pT3 or less
Pathological examination[1] of the primary carcinoma removed by short segment (limited) or radical resection with *no gross tumour* at the deep (radial, lateral), proximal and distal margins of resection (with or without microscopic involvement) *or* Pathological examination of the primary carcinoma removed by endoscopic polypectomy or local excision with histologically tumour-free margins of resection

pT4
Pathological confirmation[1] of perforation of the visceral peritoneum *or* Microscopic confirmation of invasion of adjacent organs or structures

[1]**Note.** Pathological confirmation may be achieved from biopsies or resection specimens or by cytology of specimens obtained from the serosa overlying the primary tumor (Zeng et al. 1992).

Anal Canal

pT3 or less
Pathological examination of the primary carcinoma with *no gross tumour* at the margins of resection (with or without microscopic involvement)

pT4
Microscopic confirmation of invasion of adjacent organs (e.g. vagina, urethra, bladder) (biopsy demonstration of invasion of the sphincter muscle(s) alone is not sufficient for pT4)

Liver

pT3 or less
Pathological examination of the primary carcinoma with *no gross tumour* at the margins of resection (with or without microscopic involvement)

pT4
Microscopic confirmation of multiple tumours in more than one lobe *or* Microscopic confirmation of invasion of a major branch of the portal or hepatic vein(s)

Gallbladder

pT3 or less
Pathological examination of the primary carcinoma with *no gross tumour* at the margins of resection (with or without microscopic involvement)

pT4
Microscopic confirmation of tumour in the liver more than 2 cm from the gallbladder *or* invasion of at least

two adjacent organs (stomach, duodenum, colon, pancreas, omentum, extrahepatic bile ducts, liver)

Extrahepatic Bile Ducts

pT2 or less
Pathological examination of the primary carcinoma with *no gross tumour* at the margins of resection (with or without microscopic involvement)

pT3
Microscopic confirmation of invasion of adjacent structures (liver, pancreas, duodenum, gallbladder, colon, stomach)

Ampulla of Vater

pT3 or less
Pathological examination of the primary carcinoma with *no gross tumour* at the margins of resection (with or without microscopic involvement)

pT4
Microscopic confirmation of tumour in the pancreas more than 2 cm from the ampulla *or* invasion of other adjacent organs

Pancreas

pT2 or less
Pathological examination of the primary carcinoma with *no gross tumour* at the margins of resection (with or without microscopic involvement)

pT3
Microscopic confirmation of invasion of stomach, spleen, colon and/or adjacent large vessels

pN – Regional Lymph Nodes

Site   Recommedations

Oesophagus

pN0
Histological examination of a mediastinal lymphadenectomy specimen which will ordinarily include 6 or more lymph nodes

pN1
Microscopic confirmation of at least one regional lymph node metastasis

Stomach

pN0
Histological examination of a regional lymphadenectomy specimen which will ordinarily include 15 or more lymph nodes[1]

pN1

Microscopic confirmation of metastasis in perigastric node(s) within 3 cm of the edge of the primary tumours[2]

pN2

Microscopic confirmation of metastasis in perigastric lymph node(s) more than 3 cm from the edge of the primary tumor or of metastasis in lymph node(s) along the left gastric, common hepatic, splenic or coeliac arteries

Notes. 1. Data on the number of regional lymph nodes in the upper abdomen have been reported by Wagner et al. (1991). Data from the ECC (Hermanek 1991) show that with an increasing number of examined regional lymph nodes a higher incidence of proven node-positive cases and also a higher 5-year survival rate are observed. For details see Appendix 1 on p. 68.
2. If metastases are in isolated perigastric nodes and the distance from the edge of the primary is not specified by the surgeon, classify pN1.

Small Intestine

pN0

Histological examination of a regional lymphadenectomy specimen which will ordinarily include 6 regional lymph nodes

pN1

Microscopic confirmation of regional lymph node metastasis

Colon and Rectum

pN0

Histological examination of a regional lymphadenectomy specimen which will ordinarily include 12 regional lymph nodes

pN1/2

If the pathology report does not indicate the number of involved nodes or their localization, classify pN1

pN3

Microscopic confirmation of a metastasis in a node along the course of a named vascular trunk. The "apical node" in radical resection specimens can be considered the equivalent of one on a named vascular trunk

Note. For colorectal carcinoma, the International Documentation System (Fielding et al. 1991) contains the following recommendation: "Before deeming a radical resection to be without lymph node metastasis, it is recommended that at least 12 lymph nodes be examined ... The Working Party recognized, however, that not all specimens will contain this number of lymph nodes, and this is particularly true of the patients who have received pre-operative irradiation". This recommendation is based on the data of Scott and Grace (1989) and of the SGCRC. For details see Appendix 2 on pp. 69 and 70.

Anal Canal

pN0
Histological examination of a regional perirectal – pelvic lymphadenectomy specimen which will ordinarily include 12 or more lymph nodes and/or histological examination of inguinal lymphadenectomy specimen which will ordinarily include 6 or more lymph nodes

pN1
Microscopic confirmation of metastasis in perirectal lymph node(s)

pN2
Microscopic confirmation of metastasis in internal iliac lymph node(s) of one side and/or in inguinal lymph node(s) of one side

pN3
Microscopic confirmation of metastasis in perirectal and inguinal lymph nodes, or bilateral internal iliac lymph nodes or bilateral inguinal lymph nodes

Liver

pN0
Histological examination of a regional lymphadenectomy specimen which will ordinarily include 3 or more lymph nodes

pN1
Microscopic confirmation of regional lymph node metastasis

Gallbladder,
Extrahepatic Bile Ducts

pN0
Histological examination of a lymphadenectomy specimen which will ordinarily include 3 or more lymph nodes

pN1
Microscopic confirmation of metastasis in lymph node(s) of the hepatoduodenal ligament (cystic duct, pericholedochal, hilar lymph nodes)

pN2
Microscopic confirmation of metastasis in peripancreatic (head only), periduodenal, periportal, coeliac and/or superior mesenteric lymph node(s)

Ampulla of Vater,
Pancreas

pN0
Histological examination of a regional lymphadenectomy specimen which will ordinarily include 10 or more regional lymph nodes

pN1
Microscopic confirmation of regional lymph node metastasis

Lung and Pleural Tumours

pT-Primary Tumour

Site   Recommendations

Lung Tumours   **pT3 or less**
Pathological examination of the primary carcinoma with *no gross tumour* at the margins of resection (with or without microscopic involvement)

pT4
Microscopic confirmation of invasion of any of the following: mediastinum, heart, great vessels, trachea, oesophagus, vertebral body, carina *or* Malignant cells in pleural effusion confirmed by cytology

Pleural Mesothelioma   **pT3 or less**
Pathological examination of the primary carcinoma with *no gross tumour* at the margins of resection (with or without microscopic involvement)

pT4
Microscopic confirmation of invasion of any of the following: contralateral pleura, contralateral lung, peritoneum, intra-abdominal organs, cervical tissues

pN – Regional Lymph Nodes

Site   Recommendations

Lung Tumours and   **pN0**
Pleural Mesothelioma   Histological examination of a mediastinal lymphadenectomy specimen which will ordinarily include 6 or more lymph nodes

pN1
Microscopic confirmation of metastasis in ipsilateral peribronchial lymph node(s) or ipsilateral hilar lymph node(s)

pN2
Microscopic confirmation of metastasis in ipsilateral mediastinal lymph node(s) or subcarinal lymph node(s)

pN3
Microscopic confirmation of metastasis in contralateral mediastinal lymph node(s) or contralateral hilar lymph node(s) or scalene or supraclavicular lymph node(s) (ipsilateral or contralateral)

Tumours of Bone and Soft Tissues

pT – Primary Tumour

Site	Recommendations
Bone	**pT1** Pathological examination of the primary tumour with *no gross tumour* at the margins of resection (with or without microscopic involvement) **pT2** Microscopic confirmation of invasion beyond the cortex
Soft Tissues	**pT1 and pT2** Pathological examination of the primary tumour with *no gross tumour* at the margins of resection (with or without microscopic involvement)

pN – Regional Lymph Nodes

Site	Recommendations
Bone and Soft Tissues	**pN0** Histological examination of a regional lymphadenectomy specimen which will ordinarily include 6 or more lymph nodes **pN1** Microscopic confirmation of regional lymph node metastasis

Skin Tumours

pT – Primary Tumour

Tumour type	Recommendations
Carcinoma	**pT3 or less** Pathological examination of the primary carcinoma with *no gross tumour* at the margins of resection (with or without microscopic involvement)

pT4
Microscopic confirmation of invasion of deep extra-dermal structures, i.e. cartilage, skeletal muscle or bone

Malignant Melanoma   **pT3 or less**
Pathological examination of the primary melanoma with *no gross tumour* at the lateral margins of resection *and* with no histological tumour at the deep margins of resection

pT4
Pathological examination of the primary melanoma incompletely removed but more than 4 mm in thickness and/or with invasion of the subcutaneous tissue *or* Microscopic confirmation of satellites (pT4b)

pN – Regional Lymph Nodes

Tumour type   Recommendations

Carcinoma   **pN0**
Histological examination of a regional lymphadenectomy specimen which will ordinarily include 6 or more lymph nodes

pN1
Microscopic confirmation of regional lymph node metastasis

Malignant Melanoma   **pN0**
Histological examination of a regional lymphadenectomy specimen which will ordinarily include 6 or more lymph nodes[1]

pN1
Histological examination of or positive biopsy from a regional lymph node metastasis 3 cm or less in greatest dimension[2]

pN2a
Histological examination of or positive biopsy from a regional lymph node metastasis more than 3 cm in greatest dimension

pN2b
Microscopic confirmation of an in-transit metastasis

pN2c
Both pN2a and pN2b

Notes. 1. Unpublished data from the ECC (period 1980–1986) show a relationship between the number of examined lymph nodes and pN classification. For details see Appendix 3 on p. 70.
2. If the size of the biopsied lymph node(s) is not indicated by the submitting surgeon, classify a positive biopsy from a lymph node as pN1.

Breast Tumours

pT – Primary Tumour

All pT
Recommendation: Pathological examination of the primary carcinoma with *no gross tumour* at the margins of resection (with or without microscopic involvement)

pN – Regional Lymph Nodes

Recommendations:

pN0 and pN1
Histological examination of at least the low axillary lymph nodes (Level I) which will ordinarily include 6 or more lymph nodes

pN2
Microscopic confirmation of a metastasis to ipsilateral axillary lymph nodes fixed to one another or to other structures

pN3
Microscopic confirmation of a metastasis to ipsilateral internal mammary lymph node(s)

Note. Based on the results of histological examination of 1446 patients with complete axillary dissection (Veronesi et al. 1990), a mathematical model was developed by Kiricuta and Tausch (1992) to determine the sample size from level I necessary for 90 % certainty of N0 axillary status. According to this model the examination of 10 lymph nodes from level I is needed.

Gynaecological Tumours

pT – Primary Tumours

Site	Recommendations
Vulva	**pT3 or less** Pathological examination of the primary carcinoma with *no gross tumour* at the margins of resection (with or without microscopic involvement)

pT4
Microscopic confirmation of invasion of any of the following: bladder mucosa, rectal mucosa, upper urethral mucosa, pelvic bone

Vagina

pT3 or less
Pathological examination of the primary carcinoma with *no gross tumour* at the margins of resection (with or without microscopic involvement)

pT4
Microscopic confirmation of invasion of the mucosa of bladder or rectum or of extension beyond the true pelvis

Cervix Uteri and
Corpus Uteri

pT3 or less
Pathological examination of the primary carcinoma with *no gross tumour* at the margins of resection (with or without microscopic involvement)

pT4
Microscopic confirmation of invasion of mucosa of bladder or bowel or (for cervix uteri) beyond the true pelvis

Ovary

pT1
Pathological examination of both ovaries

pT2
Microscopic confirmation of tumour outside the ovary within the pelvis *or* Cytologically proven malignant cells in ascites or peritoneal washing

pT3
Microscopic confirmation of peritoneal metastasis outside the pelvis

Note. In case of histologically proven tumour on pelvic peritoneum only but macroscopic finding of peritoneal metastasis outside the pelvis by the surgeon, the tumour is classified (c)T3pT2.

pN – Primary Tumour

Site

Recommendations

Vulva, Vagina
(Lower Third)

pN0
Histological examination of an inguinal lymphadenectomy specimen which will ordinarily include 6 or more lymph nodes

pN1
Microscopic confirmation of a unilateral regional lymph node metastasis

	pN2 Microscopic confirmation of bilateral regional lymph node metastasis
Vagina (Upper Two Thirds), Cervix Uteri, Corpus Uteri, Ovary	**pN0** Histological examination of a pelvic lymphadenectomy specimen which will ordinarily include 10 or more lymph nodes
	pN1 Microscopic confirmation of regional lymph node metastasis

Urological Tumours

pT – Primary Tumour

Site	Recommendations
Penis	**pT3 or less** Pathological examination of the primary carcinoma removed by partial or total penis amputation with *no gross tumour* at the margins of resection (with or without microscopic involvement) *or* Pathological examination of the primary tumour removed by local excision with histologically tumour-free margins of resection
	pT4 Microscopic confirmation of invasion of adjacent structures other than urethra or prostate
Prostate	**pT3 or less** Pathological examination of a radical prostatectomy specimen with *no gross tumour* at the margins of resection (with or without microscopic involvement) *or* Pathological examination of a simple prostatectomy specimen with histologically tumour-free margins of resection
	pT4 Microscopic confirmation of invasion of adjacent structures other than seminal vesicles (e. g. rectum)
Testis	**All pT** Pathological examination of a radical orchiectomy specimen

Kidney	**pT3 or less** Pathological examination of a partial or total nephrectomy specimen with *no gross tumour* at the margins of resection (with or without microscopic involvement) **pT4** Microscopic confirmation of invasion beyond Gerota fascia
Renal Pelvis and Ureter	**pT3 or less** Pathological examination of the primary carcinoma with *no gross tumour* at the margins of resection (with or without microscopic involvement) **pT4** Microscopic confirmation of invasion of perinephric fat or adjacent organs
Urinary Bladder	**pT3 or less** Pathological examination of partial or total cystectomy specimen with *no gross tumour* at the margins of resection (with or without microscopic involvement) **pT4** Microscopic confirmation of invasion of any of the following: prostate, uterus, vagina, pelvic wall, abdominal wall, intestine
Urethra	**pT3 or less** Pathological examination of the primary carcinoma with *no gross tumour* at the margins of resection (with or without microscopic involvement) **pT4** Microscopic confirmation of invasion of adjacent organs other than prostate, anterior vagina and bladder neck

pN – Regional Lymph Nodes

Site	Recommendations
All sites except penis	**pN0** Histological examination of a regional lymphadenectomy specimen which will ordinarily include 8 or more lymph nodes **pN1** Microscopic confirmation of a single lymph node metastasis not more than 2 cm in greatest dimension

pN2
Microscopic confirmation of a single lymph node metastasis more than 2 cm but not more than 5 cm in greatest dimension *or* Microscopic confirmation of at least two lymph node metastasis none more than 5 cm in greatest dimension

pN3
Microscopic confirmation of a lymph node metastasis more than 5 cm in greatest dimension

Note. Measurements are made of the metastasis not of the entire lymph node. If the size of *biopsied* lymph node(s) is not indicated by the submitting surgeon, classifiy in case of positive biopsy from one lymph node pN1 and in case of positive biopsies from two or more lymph nodes pN2.

Penis

pN0
Histological examination of an inguinal lymphadenectomy specimen which will ordinarily include 6 or more lymph nodes

pN1
Microscopic confirmation of metastasis in a single superficial inguinal lymph node

pN2
Microscopic confirmation of metastasis in multiple or bilateral superficial inguinal lymph nodes

pN3
Microscopic confirmation of metastasis in deep inguinal or pelvic lymph node(s)

Ophthalmic Tumours

pT – Primary Tumour

Site/Type

Recommendations

Carcinoma of Eyelid

pT 3 or less
Pathological examination of the primary carcinoma with histologically tumour-free margins of resection

pT4
Microscopic confirmation of invasion of adjacent structures

Malignant Melanoma of Eyelid

See Malignant Melanoma of Skin, p. 59

Carcinoma of Conjunctiva	**pT 3 or less** Pathological examination of the primary carcinoma with histologically tumour-free margins of resection **pT4** Microscopic confirmation of invasion of the orbit
Malignant Melanoma of Conjunctiva	**pT3 or less** Pathological examination of the primary melanoma with histologically tumour-free margins of resection **pT4** Microscopic confirmation of invasion of the eyelid, cornea and/or orbit
Malignant Melanoma of Uvea	**pT3 or less** Pathological examination of the primary melanoma with histologically tumour-free margins of resection **pT4** Microscopic confirmation of extraocular extension
Retinoblastoma	**pT3 or less** Pathological examination of the primary retinoblastoma with histologically tumour-free margins of resection **pT4** Microscopic confirmation of tumour at the line of resection or other extraocular extension
Sarcoma of Orbit	**pT3 or less** Pathological examination of the primary sarcoma with histologically tumour-free margins of resection **pT4** Microscopic confirmation of tumour beyond the orbit (adjacent sinuses and/or cranium)
Carcinoma of Lacrimal Gland	**pT3 or less** Pathological examination of the primary carcinoma with *no gross tumour* at the margins of resection (with or without microscopic involvement) **pT4** Microscopic confirmation of bone invasion

pN – Regional Lymph Nodes

Site	Recommendations
All Sites and Types	**pN0** Histological examination of a regional lymphadenectomy specimen which will ordinarily include 6 or more lymph nodes **pN1** Microscopic confirmation of regional lymph node metastasis

Brain Tumours

pT – Primary Tumour

Site	Recommendations
Supratentorial	**pT3 or less** Pathological examination of the primary tumour with *no gross tumour* at the margins of resection (with or without microscopic involvement) **pT4** Microscopic confirmation of tumour beyond the midline of brain, in the opposite hemisphere and/or infratentorially
Infratentorial	**pT3 or less** Pathological examination of the primary tumour with *no gross tumour* at the margins of resection (with or without microscopic involvement) **pT4** Microscopic confirmation of tumour beyond the midline of brain, in the opposite hemisphere and/or supratentorially

Hodgkin Disease and Non-Hodgkin Lymphomas

Pathological staging requires the histological examination of:

- Liver biopsies
- At least 4 abdominal lymph nodes
- Marrow biopsies
- Spleen or spleen biopsies

Paediatric Tumours

pT – Primary Tumour

All Sites and Types

pT3b or less
Pathological examination of the resected primary tumour

pT3c and 4
Surgical exploration without tumour resection

pN – Primary Tumour

All Sites and Types

pN0
Histological examination of a regional lymphadenectomy specimen which will ordinarily include 3 or more lymph nodes

pN1
Microscopic confirmation of regional lymph node metastasis and surgical statements on completeness of resection

Appendix 1. Stomach Carcinoma

The data in Tables 3 and 4 are from the ECC (Hermanek 1991), and concern only patients with radical resection for cure (RO).

Table 3. Number of regional lymph nodes examined and pN classification

Number of regional lymph nodes examined	Number of patients	Patients with histologically proven regional lymph node metastasis (pN1, 2)	
		(n)	(%)
≤ 5	11	2	18
6–15	48	14	29
16–25	93	42	45
26–35	149	82	55.0
36–45	132	78	59.1
> 45	278	184	66.2

Table 4. Prognosis in relation to number of regional lymph nodes examined (patients operated on 1978–1989, those with extended surgery excluded)

Patient group	Number of patients	5-year survival rate with standard error (%)[a]	
		Observed	Relative
Total gastrectomy			
1–25 nodes examined	18	28 ± 10	33 ± 13
> 25 nodes examined	122	47 ± 5	56 ± 6
Subtotal gastrectomy			
1–15 nodes examined	43	51 ± 8	71 ± 11
16–25 nodes examined	48	57 ± 8	71 ± 10
1–25 nodes examined	91	54 ± 6	71 ± 7
> 25 nodes examined	121	68 ± 5	83 ± 6

[a] Kaplan Meier, surgical mortality not excluded.
Differences between ≤ 25 and > 25: $p = 0.05 - 0.10$

Appendix 2. Colorectal Carcinoma

The data of the SGCRC on pN classification in relation to the number of regional lymph nodes examined are shown in Figs. 12 and 13 separately for rectum and colon carcinoma treated by radical resection for cure (R0). In Fig. 14 data for both carcinomas are combined and divided according to the R classification. A summary of preliminary data was published by Hermanek (1991).

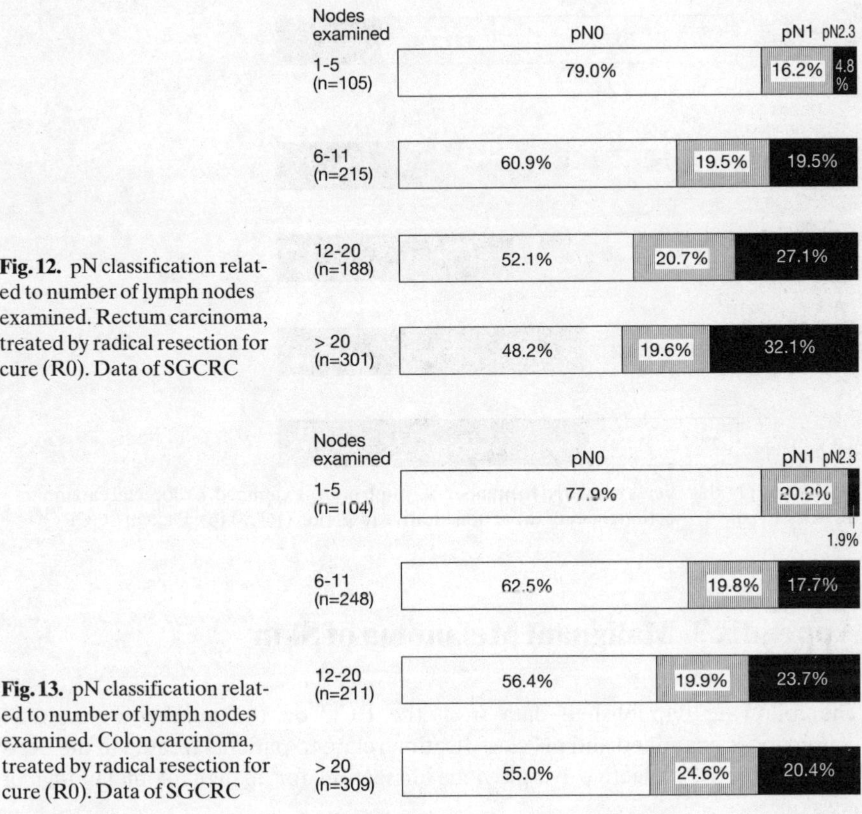

Fig. 12. pN classification related to number of lymph nodes examined. Rectum carcinoma, treated by radical resection for cure (R0). Data of SGCRC

Fig. 13. pN classification related to number of lymph nodes examined. Colon carcinoma, treated by radical resection for cure (R0). Data of SGCRC

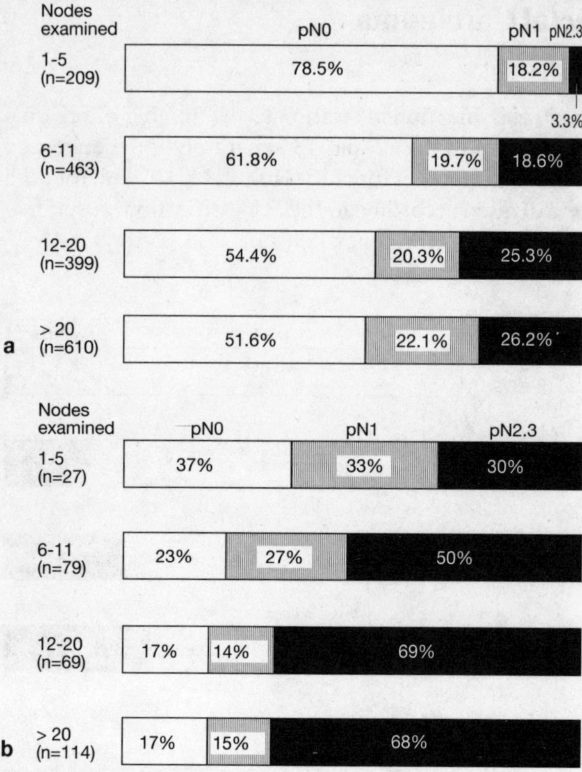

Fig. 14a, b. pN classification related to number of lymph nodes examined. Colorectal carcinoma, treated by radical resection for cure **(a)** or noncurative resection (R1, 2) **(b)**. Data of SGCRC

Appendix 3. Malignant Melanoma of Skin

The following unpublished data from the ECC on the number of regional lymph nodes examined and pN classification relate to patients treated in the period 1980–1986 by elective lymph node dissection for malignant melanoma of the skin.

Table 5. Number of regional lymph nodes examined and pN classification

Number of lymph nodes examined	Number of patients	Patients with regional lymph node metastasis (n)	(%)
1–5	22	0	
6–15	122	11	9.8
16–25	83	12	14
> 25	28	3	11

References

Fielding LP, Arsenault PA, Chapuis PH, Dent O, Gatright B, Hardcastle JD, Hermanek P, Jass JR, Newland RC (1991) Clinicopathological staging for colorectal cancer: an International Documentation System (IDS) and an International Comprehensive Anatomical Terminology (ICAT). J Gastroenterol Hepatol 6: 325–344

Hermanek P (1991) Onkologische Chirurgie/Pathologisch-anatomische Sicht. Langenbecks Arch Chir Suppl 277–281

Hermanek P, Giedl J, Dworak O (1989) Two programmes for examination of regional lymph nodes in colorectal carcinoma with regard to the new pN classification. Pathol Res Pract 185: 867–873

Honthoff MJ (1989) Surgical pathology of hepatobiliary and pancreatic tumours. In: Lygidakis NJ, Tytgat GNJ (eds) Hepatobiliary and pancreatic malignancies. Thieme, Stuttgart

Kiricuta Cl, Tausch J (1992) A mathematical model of axillary lymph node involvement based on 1446 complete axillary dissections in patients with breast carcinoma. Cancer 69: 2496–2501

Qizilbash AH (1982) Pathologic studies in colorectal cancer. Pathol Annu 17: 1–46

Remmele W (1984) Staging, typing and grading of colorectal cancer: a critical review of current classification systems. Prog Surg Pathol 5: 7–36

Robbins KT, Medina JE, Wolfe GT, Levine PA, Sessions RB, Pruet CW (1991) Standardizing neck dissection terminology. Official report of the Academy's Committee for Head and Neck Surgery and Oncology. Arch Otolaryngol Head Neck Surg 117: 601–605

Rosai J (1989) Ackerman's surgical pathology, 7th edn. Mosby, St. Louis

Scott KWM, Grace RH (1989) Detection of lymph node metastases in colorectal carcinoma before and after fat clearance. Br J Surg 76: 1165–1167

Veronesi U, Luini A, Galimberti V, Marchini S, Sacchini V, Rilke F (1990) Extent of metastatic axillary involvement in 1446 cases of breast cancer. Eur J Surg Oncol 16: 127–133

Wagner PK, Ramaswamy A, Rüschoff J, Schmitz-Moormann P, Rothmund M (1991) Lymph node counts in the upper abdomen: anatomical basis for lymphadenectomy in gastric cancer. Br J Surg 78: 825–827

Zeng Z, Cohen AM, Hajdu S, Sternberg SS, Sigurdson ER, Enker W (1992) Serosal cytologic study to determine free mesothelial penetration by intraperitoneal colon cancer. Cancer 70: 737–740

New Classifications
Recommended for Testing

Introduction

This chapter contains proposals for new classifications as follows:

1. Nasal cavity and paranasal sinus (other than maxillary sinus)
2. Gastrointestinal sarcomas
3. Malignant Thymoma
4. Cranial and facial bones
5. Cutaneous T-cell lymphoma
6. Fallopian tube
7. Gestational trophoblastic tumours
8. Chronic myeloid leukaemia
9. Primary liver carcinoma in infants and children

These new classifications are provisional. Testing by several institutions and on larger numbers of patients is needed before general acceptance can be recommended. Those having relevant data, published or not, on these classifications are invited to contact the TNM Project Committee of the UICC through their national TNM Committees or any of the editors of this publication.

Nasal Cavity and Paranasal Sinus (Other Than Maxillary Sinus) (ICD-O C30.0, 31.1,2,3)

The following classification, which applies to carcinomas, was proposed by Schwab et al. (1988).

Anatomical Sites and Subsites

1. Nasal cavity[1]
   a) Inferior wall
   b) Superior wall including the superior nasal concha
   c) Lateral wall including the middle and inferior nasal concha
   d) Medial wall
2. Upper region of paranasal sinuses
   a) Maxilloethmoidal angle
   b) Ethmoidal sinus
   c) Sphenoid sinus
   d) Frontal sinus
3. Maxillary Sinus
4. Adjacent sites
   a) Oral cavity mucosa, upper alveolus and gingiva and/or hard palate
   b) Orbit

Note. 1. Anterior border, vestibulum nasi; posterior border, margin of the choanal orifices and posterior margin of the nasal septum.

TNM Clinical Classification

T – Primary Tumour

TX   Primary tumour cannot be assessed
T0   No evidence of primary tumour
Tis   Carcinoma in situ

T1   Tumour limited to one subsite
T2   Tumour limited to one site
T3   Tumour invades 2 or 3 sites or one of the adjacent sites
T4   Tumour invades both adjacent sites or other structures, e.g. skin, ptery-gopalatine fossa, base of the skull, cranial fossa, endocranium, frontal bone, nasopharynx, infratemporal fossa

N – Regional Lymph Nodes

As in other head and neck tumours.

M – Distant Metastasis

As in other head and neck tumours.

Stage Grouping

Stage 0	Tis	N0	M0
Stage I	T1	N0	M0
Stage II	T2	N0	M0
Stage III	T1	N1	M0
	T2	N1	M0
	T3	N0, N1	M0
Stage IV	T4	N0, N1	M0
	Any T	N2, N3	M0
	Any T	Any N	M1

Note. The stage grouping corresponds to that for maxillary sinus.

Supporting Data

The German Working Group on Head and Neck Surgery (AO/HNO) presented the following survival data for 1546 patients, including those with maxillary sinus tumours (Schwab 1990):

	Frequency (%)	Cumulative 5 year survival rates (%) (actuarial method)
T1	9	(80) (small number of patients)
T2	20	48
T3	30	23
T4	38	12
TX	3	

Addendum
1. Dr. Badellino presented the following proposal of Prof. Calearo for nasal cavity and paranasal sinus in 1990:
TX, T0, Tis as usual
T1   Tumour limited to one site without bone invasion
T2   Tumour limited to one site with bone involvement
T3   Tumour involves 2 or more sites but does not extend beyond
T4   Tumour extends beyond the sites, e.g. involves oral cavity, orbit, base of the skull, nasopharynx, skin, pterygomaxillary fossa
Sites: Nasal cavity
       Maxillary sinus
       Ethmoid sinus
       Frontal sinus
       Sphenoid sinus
Supporting data are not available, and so the German proposal is recommended.
2. The SEER Program staging system for paranasal sinus (other than maxillary) is not recommended because it is not applicable to carcinomas of the nasal cavity.

Gastrointestinal Sarcomas
(ICD-O C15–C21)

The classification is based on preliminary data from the SEER Program suggesting the use of the present classification of soft tissue sarcomas for visceral sarcomas.

Rules for Classification

The classification applies to sarcomas of gastrointestinal hollow viscera. Kaposi sarcoma is not included. There should be histological confirmation of the disease. The cases should be recorded by histological type and grade.

The following are the procedures for assessing the T, N and M categories:

T categories   Physical examination and imaging
N categories   Physical examination and imaging
M categories   Physical examination and imaging

Anatomical Sites

1. Oesophagus (C15)
2. Stomach (C16)
3. Small intestine (C17)
4. Colon (C18)
5. Rectum (including rectosigmoid junction) (C19, C20)
6. Anal Canal (C21.1,2)

Regional Lymph Nodes

The regional lymph nodes are those appropriate to the site of the primary tumour.

TNM Clinical Classification

T – Primary Tumour

TX   Primary tumour cannot be assessed
T0   No evidence of primary tumour

T1   Tumour 5 cm or less in greatest dimension
T2   Tumour more than 5 cm in greatest dimension

N – Regional Lymph Nodes

NX   Regional lymph nodes cannot be assessed
N0   No regional lymph node metastasis
N1   Regional lymph node metastasis

M – Distant Metastasis

MX   Presence of distant metastasis cannot be assessed
M0   No distant metastasis
M1   Distant metastasis

pTNM Pathological Classification

The pT, pN and pM categories correspond to the T, N and M categories.

G Histopathological Grading

GX   Grade of differentiation cannot be assessed
G1   Well differentiated
G2   Moderately differentiated
G3   Poorly differentiated
G4   Undifferentiated

Note. After the histological type has been determined, the tumour should be graded according to
the accepted criteria including particularly mitotic activity but also cellularity, cellular pleomorphism and necrosis.

Stage Grouping

Stage IA	G1	T1	N0	M0
Stage IB	G1	T2	N0	M0
Stage IIA	G2	T1	N0	M0
Stage IIB	G2	T2	N0	M0
Stage IIIA	G3, 4	T1	N0	M0
Stage IIIB	G3, 4	T2	N0	M0
Stage IVA	Any G	Any T	N1	M0
Stage IVB	Any G	Any T	Any N	M1

Summary

Gastrointestinal Sarcomas	
T1	$\leqslant 5$ cm
T2	> 5 cm
N1	Regional
G1	Well differentiated
G2	Moderately differentiated
G3	Poorly differentiated
G4	Undifferentiated

Malignant Thymoma
(ICD-O C37)

The classification is based on Japanese data published by Yamakawa et al. (1991).

Rules for Classification

The classification applies to malignant thymoma, i. e. malignant epithelial tumour originating from thymus gland (Rosai and Levine 1976), and to thymic carcinoid tumours. Germinal tumour and malignant lymphoma are excluded from this classification even if they originate from thymus.

The following are the procedures for assessing the T, N and M categories:

T categories   Physical examination and imaging, endoscopy and/or surgical exploration
N categories   Physical examination and imaging, endoscopy and/or surgical exploration
M categories   Physical examination and imaging and/or surgical exploration

Regional Lymph Nodes

The regional lymph nodes are the intrathoracic, scalene and supraclavicular nodes.

TNM Clinical Classification

T – Primary Tumour

TX   Primary tumour cannot be assessed
T0   No evidence of primary tumour

T1   Completely encapsulated tumour
T2   Invasion of pericapsular connective tissue
T3   Invasion into neighbouring structures, such as pericardium, mediastinal pleura, thorax wall, great vessels and lung
T4   Pleural or pericardial dissemination

N – Regional Lymph Nodes

NX   Regional lymph nodes cannot be assessed
N0   No regional lymph node metastasis
N1   Metastasis in anterior mediastinal lymph nodes
N2   Metastasis in other intrathoracic lymph nodes
N3   Metastasis in scalene and/or supraclavicular lymph nodes

M – Distant Metastasis

MX   Presence of distant metastasis cannot be assessed
M0   No distant metastasis
M1   Distant metastasis

pTNM Pathological Classification

The pT, pN and pM categories correspond to the T, N and M categories.

Stage Grouping

Stage I	T1	N0	M0
Stage II	T2	N0	M0
Stage III	T1	N1	M0
	T2	N1	M0
	T3	N0, 1	M0
Stage IV	T4	Any N	M0
	Any T	N2, 3	M0
	Any T	Any N	M1

Summary

Thymus	
T1	Completely encapsulated
T2	Pericapsular connective tissue
T3	Neighbouring structures, e. g. pericardium, mediastinal pleura, thorax wall, great vessels, lung
T4	Pleural/pericardial dissemination
N1	Anterior mediastinal
N2	Other intrathoracic
N3	Scalene/supraclavicular

Cranial and Facial Bones
(ICD-O C41.0,1)

The classification is based on the results of a field trial carried out by B. Spiessl, Basel, Switzerland, and W. Piotrowski, Mannheim, Germany, on behalf of the DSK-TNM from 1974 to 1988. The study includes 351 patients with malignant tumours (see supporting data, p. 83).

Rules for Classification

There should be histological classification of the disease to permit division of cases by histological type which is needed for the T classification.

The following are the procedures for assessment of the T, N and M categories:

T categories   Physical examination and imaging
N categories   Physical examination and imaging
M categories   Physical examination and imaging

Anatomical Subsites

1. Bones of skull (C41.0): frontal bone, parietal bone, occipital bone, sphenoid bone, temporal bone
2. Bones of face (C41.0): ethmoid bone, inferior nasal concha, lacrimal bone, maxillary bone, nasal bone, palatine bone, vomer, zygomatic bone
3. Mandible (C41.1)

Histological Types of Tumours

The following histological types of malignant tumours are included, the appropriate ICD-O morphology rubrics being indicated:

1. Osteosarcomas (9180–9190/3)
2. Other sarcomas:
   a) Malignant fibrous tumours
      Fibrosarcoma (8810/3)
      Fibromyxosarcoma (8811/3)
      Fibrous histiocytoma, malignant (8830/3)
   b) Malignant blood vessel tumours
      Hemangiosarcoma (9120/3)
      Hemangioendothelioma, malignant (9130/3)
      Epithelioid hemangioendothelioma, malignant (9133/3)
      Hemangiopericytoma, malignant (9150/3)
   c) Malignant chondromatous tumours
      Chondrosarcoma (9220/3)
      Chondroblastoma, malignant (9230/3)
      Myxoid chondrosarcoma (9231/3)
      Mesenchymal chondrosarcoma (9240/3)
   d) Malignant odontogenic tumours (9270/3–9330/3)
   e) Malignant nerve sheath tumours
      Neurofibrosarcoma (9540/3)
      Neurilemmoma, malignant (9560/3)

Regional Lymph Nodes

The regional lymph nodes are the preauricular, submandibular and cervical lymph nodes.

TNM Clinical Classification

T – Primary Tumour

TX   Primary tumour cannot be assessed
T0   No evidence of primary tumour

Osteosarcomas
T1   Tumour limited to mandible
      T1a Tumour confined within the cortex
      T1b Tumour invades beyond the cortex

T2   Tumour limited to bones of face
      T2a Well delimited tumour
      T2b Poorly delimited tumour
T3   Tumour limited to bones of skull
      T3a Tumour confined within the cortex
      T3b Tumour invades beyond the cortex
T4   Tumour involves more than one subsite

Other Sarcomas
T1   Tumour 4 cm or less in greatest dimension
      T1a Well delimited tumour
      T1b Poorly delimited tumour
T2   Tumour more than 4 cm in greatest dimension
      T2a Well delimited tumour
      T2b Poorly delimited tumour

Note. The subdivisions into a and b are optional.
      Tumours which are partly well, partly poorly delimited are classified as poorly delimited.

N – Regional Lymph Nodes

NX   Regional lymph nodes cannot be assessed
N0   No regional lymph node metastasis
N1   Regional lymph node metastasis

M – Distant Metastasis

MX   Presence of distant metastasis cannot be assessed
M0   No distant metastasis
M1   Distant metastasis

pTNM Pathological Classification

The pT, pN and pM categories correspond to the T, N and M categories.

Stage Grouping

No stage grouping is at present recommended.

Summary

Cranial and Facial Bones		
	Osteosarcomas	
T1		Limited to mandible
	T1a	Within cortex
	T1b	Beyond cortex
T2		Limited to facial bones
	T2a	Well delimited
	T2b	Poorly delimited
T3		Limited to skull
	T3a	Within cortex
	T3b	Beyond cortex
T4		> One subsite
	Other Sarcomas	
T1		$\leqslant$ 4 cm
	T1a	Well delimited
	T1b	Poorly delimited
T2		> 4 cm
	T2a	Well delimited
	T2b	Poorly delimited
	All Types	
N1		Regional

Addendum

The results of the German field trial (Spiessl and Piotrowski) may be summarized as follows:

1. According to a multivariate regression analysis histology, tumour site, tumour size and delimitation are independent prognostic factors.
2. The most important prognostic factor in osteosarcoma is tumour site (Fig. 15).
3. In other sarcomas tumour size is the most important prognostic factor (Fig. 16).
4. In osteosarcoma and other sarcomas invasion beyond cortex and poor delimitation of tumour show a trend to worsening of prognosis, but statistical significance was not achieved.

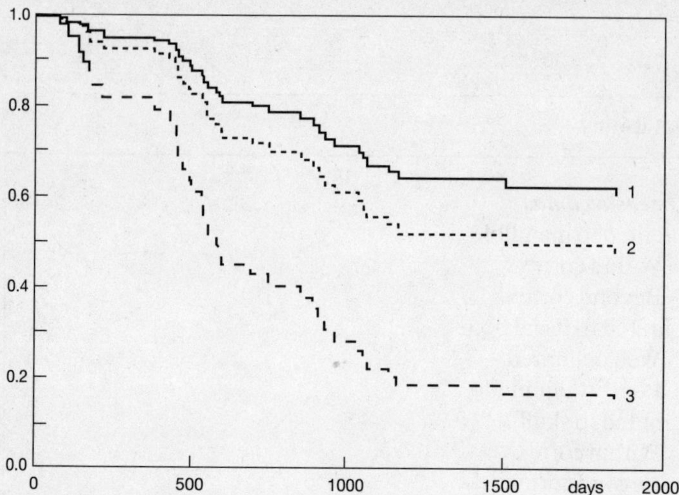

Fig. 15. Observed survival in osteosarcoma in relation to site: *1,* mandible ($n = 46$); *2,* bones of face ($n = 356$); *3,* skull ($n = 10$) ($p = 0.024$)

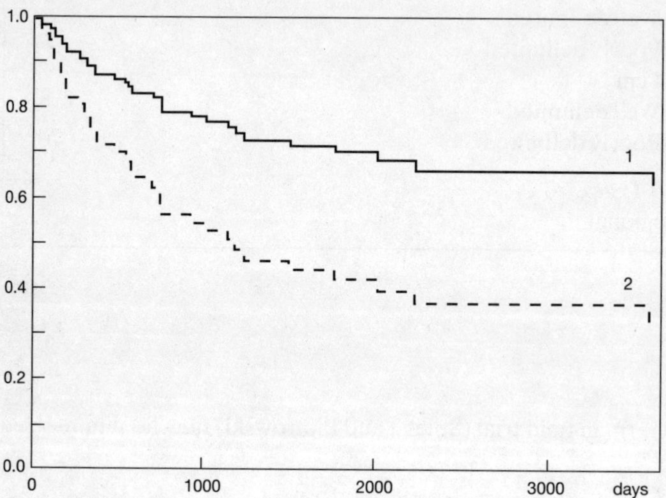

Fig. 16. Observed survival in other sarcomas in relation to size: *1,* $\leq$ 4 cm ($n = 52$); *2,* > 4 cm ($n = 34$) ($p = 0.029$)

Cutaneous T-Cell Lymphoma
(Excluding Lip, Eyelid, Vulva and Penis)
(ICD-O C44.2–7, C63.2)

A TNM classification for mycosis fungoides of the skin was proposed by the American Mycosis Fungoides Study Group in 1979 (Bunn and Lamberg 1979). It was used for T-cell lymphomas other than mycosis fungoides by the European Organization for Research and Treatment of Cancer/German Federal Ministry for Research and Technology Cutaneous Lymphoma Group (Burg et al. 1987). The N classification is not consistent with the principles of the TNM system used for other anatomical sites or entities. Therefore, in the following classification the N categories differ from those in the classification of the American Mycosis Fungoides Study Group. However, a "translation" is easily possible (see following table), and stage grouping is not influenced:

American Mycosis Fungoides Study Group	Proposed TNM
N0	N0, pN0
N1	N1, pN0
N2	N0, pN1
N3	N1, pN1

Note. The definitions of T and M and stage grouping are identical in both classifications.

Rules for Classification

The classification applies to any type of cutaneous T-cell lymphoma. There should be histological confirmation of the disease.

The following are the procedures for assessment of T, N and M categories:

T categories	Physical examination, mapping of skin lesions and skin biopsies
N categories	Physical examination, imaging and biopsy
M categories	Physical examination, imaging and biopsy (e.g. bone marrow or liver)

Anatomical Sites

The following sites are identified by the ICD-O topography rubrics:

1. External ear and other parts of face (excluding lip and eyelid) (C44.2, 3)
2. Scalp and neck (C44.4)
3. Trunk (including anal margin and perianal skin) (C44.5)

4. Arm and shoulder (C44.6)
5. Leg and hip (C44.7)
6. Scrotum (C63.2)

Regional Lymph Nodes

The regional lymph nodes are the superficial nodes, i.e. those of head and neck (preauricular, submandibular, cervical), and the axillary, epitrochlear, inguinal and popliteal nodes.

TNM Clinical Classification

T – Primary Tumour

TX   Primary tumour cannot be assessed
T0   No evidence of primary tumour

T1   Limited plaques, papules, or eczematous patches covering less than 10% of the skin surface
T2   Disseminated plaques, papules or erythematous patches covering 10% or more of the skin surface
T3   Tumour(s) (one or more)
T4   Generalized erythroderma

Note. When characteristics of more than one T category exist, the highest is used for classification.

Definitions (International League of Dermatological Societies 1987)
Plaque: Flat or elevated lesion with increased consistency
Papule: Small elevated nodular lesion 1 cm or less in greatest dimension
Patch: Change of skin colour larger than "macule" would suggest
Tumour: Nodular lesion, more than 1 cm in greatest dimension
Macule: Area of discoloration
Erythroderma: Generalized redness of skin, often combined with scaling and edema

N – Regional Lymph Nodes

NX   Regional lymph nodes cannot be assessed
N0   No involvement of regional lymph nodes
N1   Involvement of regional lymph nodes

M – Nonregional Extracutaneous Involvement ("Distant Metastasis")

MX   Nonregional extracutaneous involvement cannot be assessed
N0   No nonregional extracutaneous involvement
M1   Nonregional extracutaneous involvement

pTNM Pathological Classification

The pT, pN and pM categories correspond to the T, N and M categories.

Stage Grouping

Stage IA	T1	N0	pN0, X	M0
Stage IB	T2	N0	pN0, X	M0
Stage IIA	T1	N1	pN0, X	M0
	T2	N1	pN0, X	M0
Stage IIB	T3	Any N	pN0, X	M0
Stage III	T4	Any N	pN0, X	M0
Stage IVA	Any T	Any N	pN1	M0
Stage IVB	Any T	Any N	Any pN	M1

Note. For comparison with the original Classification of the American Mycosis Fungoides Study Group, see Introduction, p. 85.

Summary

Cutaneous T-cell Lymphoma	
T1	Limited plaques, papules or patches ($< 10\%$ of skin surface)
T2	Disseminated plaques, papules or patches ($\geqslant 10\%$ of skin surface)
T3	Tumour(s)
T4	Generalized erythroderma
N1	Regional

Fallopian Tube
(ICD-O C57.0)

The following classification for carcinoma of the fallopian tube is based on that of FIGO adopted in 1992 (Creasman 1992). The definitions of the T categories correspond to the several stages accepted by FIGO. Both systems are included for comparison.

Rules for Classification

The classification applies only to carcinoma. There should be histological confirmation of the disease.

The following are the procedures for assessing the T, N and M categories:

T categories   Physical examination, imaging, laparoscopy and/or surgical exploration

N categories   Physical examination, imaging, laparoscopy and/or surgical exploration

M categories   Physical examination, imaging, laparoscopy and/or surgical exploration

The FIGO stages are based on surgical staging. (TNM stages are based on clinical and/or pathological classification.)

Regional Lymph Nodes

The regional lymph nodes are the hypogastric (obturator), common iliac, external iliac, lateral sacral, para-aortic and inguinal nodes.

TNM Clinical Classification

T – Primary Tumour

TNM categories	*FIGO stages*		
TX			Primary tumour cannot be assessed
T0			No evidence of primary tumour
Tis	0		Carcinoma in situ
T1	I		Tumour limited to fallopian tube(s)
	T1a	IA	Tumour limited to one tube; serosa intact, no tumour on the surface of tube; no ascites
	T1b	IB	Tumour limited to both tubes; serosa intact, no tumour on the surface of tubes; no ascites
	T1c	IC	Tumour limited to one or both tube(s) with any of the following: serosa penetrated, tumour on the surface of tubes, malignant cells in ascites or peritoneal washings
T2		II	Tumour involves one or both fallopian tube(s) with pelvic extension

T2a	IIA	Extension and/or metastasis on uterus and/or ovaries
T2b	IIB	Extension to other pelvic structures[1]
T2c	IIC	Direct extension (2a or 2b) with malignant cells in ascites or peritoneal washings
T3 and/or N1	III	Tumour involves one or both fallopian tube(s) with microscopically confirmed peritoneal metastasis outside the pelvis and/or regional lymph node metastasis
T3a	IIIA	Microscopic metastasis outside the pelvis
T3b	IIIB	Macroscopic peritoneal metastasis outside the pelvis 2 cm or less in greatest dimension
T3c and/ or N1	IIIC	Peritoneal metastasis outside the pelvis more than 2 cm in greatest dimension and/or regional lymph node metastasis
M1	IV	Distant metastasis (excludes peritoneal metastasis)[2]

Notes. 1. A tumour limited to the pelvis but with histologically proven extension to the small bowel or omentum is not T2b/stage IIB, but T3a/stage IIIA.
2. Liver capsule metastasis is T3/stage III, liver parenchymal metastasis M1/stage IV. Pleural effusion must have positive cytology for M1/stage IV.

N – Regional Lymph Nodes

NX   Regional lymph nodes cannot be assessed
N0   No regional lymph node metastasis
N1   Regional lymph node metastasis

M – Distant Metastasis

MX   Presence of distant metastasis cannot be assessed
N0   No distant metastasis
M1   Distant metastasis

pTNM Pathological Classification

The pT, pN and pM categories correspond to the T, N and M categories.

G Histopathological Grading

GX   Grade cannot be assessed
GB   Borderline malignancy
G1   Well differentiated
G2   Moderately differentiated
G3–4   Poorly differentiated or undifferentiated

Stage Grouping

Stage IA	T1a	N0	M0
Stage IB	T1b	N0	M0
Stage IC	T1c	N0	M0
Stage IIA	T2a	N0	M0
Stage IIB	T2b	N0	M0
Stage IIC	T2c	N0	M0
Stage IIIA	T3a	N0	M0
Stage IIIB	T3b	N0	M0
Stage IIIC	T3c	N0	M0
	Any T	N1	M0
Stage IV	Any T	Any N	M1

Summary

TNM	*Fallopian Tube*	*FIGO*
T1	Limited to tube(s)	I
T1a	One tube, serosa intact	IA
T1b	Both tubes, serosa intact	IB
T1c	Serosa penetrated, malignant cells in ascites or peritoneal washings	IC
T2	Pelvic extension	II
T2a	Uterus, ovaries	IIA
T2b	Other pelvic structures	IIB
T2c	Malignant cells in ascites or peritoneal washings	IIC
T3 and/or N1	Peritoneal metastasis outside pelvis and/or regional lymph node metastasis	III
T3a	Microscopic peritoneal metastasis	IIIA
T3b	Macroscopic peritoneal metastasis $\leqslant$ 2 cm	IIIB
T3c and/or N1	Peritoneal metastasis > 2 cm and/or regional lymph node metastasis	IIIC
M1	Distant metastasis (excludes peritoneal metastasis)	IV

Gestational Trophoblastic Tumours (ICD-O C58.9)

The following classification for gestational trophoblastic tumours is based on that of FIGO adopted 1992 (Creasman 1992). The definitions of the T categories correspond to the several stages accepted by FIGO. Both systems are included for comparison. In stage grouping, risk factors are considered in addition to T and M. In contrast to other sites, an N classification does not apply to these tumours.

Rules for Classification

The classification applies to choriocarcinoma (9100/3), invasive hydatidiform mole (9100/1) and placental site trophoblastic tumour (9104/1). Placental site tumours should be reported separately. Histological confirmation is not required if the urine human chorionic gonadotropin (hCG) level is abnormally elevated.

The following are the procedures for assessing the T and M categories:

T categories   Physical examination, imaging including urography and cystoscopy, and urine hCG level

M categories   Physical examination, imaging and assessment of urine hCG level

Risk factors   There are two major risk factors that may affect outcome (other than T and M)
1. hCG more than 100 000 IU/24 h urine
2. Duration of disease longer than 6 months from termination of antecedent pregnancy

TM Clinical Classification

T – Primary Tumour

TM categories	FIGO stages[1]	
TX	–	Primary tumour cannot be assessed
T0	–	No evidence of primary tumour
T1	I	Tumour limited to uterus
T2	II	Tumour involves other genital structures: vagina, ovary, broad ligament, fallopian tube (by metastasis or direct extension)
M1a	III	Metastasis to the lung(s)[2]
M1b	IV	Metastasis (e. g. brain) with or without lung involvement[2]

Notes. 1. The FIGO stages I to IV are subdivided into A to C according to the number of risk factors: **A** without any risk factors, **B** with one risk factor, **C** with two risk factors.
2. Genital metastasis (vagina, ovary, broad ligament, fallopian tube) is classified T2.

M – Metastasis

MX   Presence of metastasis cannot be assessed
M0   No metastasis
M1   Metastasis
    M1a Metastasis to lung(s)
    M1b Metastasis (e. g. brain) with or without lung involvement

Note. Genital metastasis (vagina, ovary, broad ligament, fallopian tube) is classified T2.

pTM Pathological Classification

The pT and pM categories correspond to the T and M categories.

Stage Grouping

Stage		TM	Risk factors
I	A	T1M0	without
	B		one
	C		two
II	A	T2M0	without
	B		one
	C		two
III	A	Any T M1a	without
	B		one
	C		two
IV	A	Any T M1b	without
	B		one
	C		two

Summary

TM	**Gestational Trophoblastic Tumours**	*FIGO*
T1	Limited to uterus	I
T2	Other genital structures	II
M1a	Metastasis with lung(s)	III
M1b	Metastasis with or without lung involvement	IV

FIGO stages are further subdivided:
A without any risk factors
B with one risk factor
C with two risk factors

Chronic Myeloid Leukaemia

The following classification (Ross et al. 1993) has been endorsed by the AJCC and the UICC. It is based on three parameters, namely T (tumour), F (risk factors) and E (extramedullary tumour). N and M classifications do not apply to this entity.

Rules for Classification

The classification applies only to chronic myeloid leukaemia. There must be haematological confirmation of the disease.

The following are the procedures for assessing the T, F and E categories:

T categories   Blood and bone marrow examination
F categories   Platelet count, haemoglobin value, basophil count, karyotype or *bcr/abl* gene rearrangement analysis
E categories   Physical examination, imaging, histology or cytology of extramedullary site(s)

Staging Criteria

T – Tumour

T1   5 % or less blasts in bone marrow or blood
T2   More than 5 % but not more than 15 % blasts in bone marrow or blood
T3   More than 15 % but not more than 30 % blasts in bone marrow or blood
T4   More than 30 % blasts in bone marrow or blood

F – Risk Factors

The risk factors (other than T or E) that may affect outcome are:

– Platelets less than 100 k/µl
– Haemoglobin less than 7 g/dl
– Basophilia greater than 20 %
– Karyotypic evolution

F0   No risk factor
F1   One risk factor
F2   More than one risk factor

E – Extramedullary Tumour

E0   No extramedullary tumour, or tumour with 30 % or less blasts in an extramedullary site
E1   Tumour with more than 30 % blasts in an extramedullary site

Stage Grouping

Phase	Stage			
Chronic	IA	T1	F0	E0
	IB	T2	F0	E0
Accelerated	IIA	TI	FI	E0
		T1	F2	E0
		T2	F1	E0
	IIB	T2	F2	E0
		T3	Any F	E0
Blastic (acute)	IIIA	T4	Any F	E0
	IIIB	Any T	Any F	E1

Summary

Chronic Myeloid Leukaemia	
T1	$\leq 5\%$ blasts
T2	$> 5\%$ to 15% blasts
T3	$> 15\%$ to 30% blasts
T4	$> 30\%$ blasts
F0	No risk factor
F1	One risk factor
F2	More than one risk factor
E0	No extramedullary tumour or extramedullary tumour $\leq 30\%$ blasts
E1	Extramedullary tumour $> 30\%$ blasts

Definitions and Explanatory Notes

Definitions

Chronic myeloid leukaemia (CML) is a haematopoietic malignancy characterized by an increase in peripheral blood cell counts, bone marrow hypercellularity and a *bcr/abl* gene fusion detected either by molecular techniques or by karyotypic analysis for the Philadelphia chromosome. Other myeloproliferative syndromes such as essential thrombocytosis which are positive for *bcr/abl* will be considered as CML. So-called atypical CML and juvenile CML which are negative for *bcr/abl* will be treated as a non-CML myelodysplastic syndrome. Thus, CML may be considered as one of the first diseases essentially to be defined by the presence of an acquired gene defect which is best detected by molecular diagnostics. This gene defect, the fusion of the *bcr* gene on chromosome 22 with the *abl* oncogene from chromosome 9, was recognized as an abnormal chromosomal translocation, the Philadelphia chromosome, years before the development of recombinant DNA technology. Research, including transgenic mouse models of CML, has shown that the *bcr/abl* fusion gene produces an abnormal protein which is related to the pathogenesis of the bone marrow neoplastic proliferation.

Clinical

CML may have a prolonged unrecognized preclinical stage. The disease usually presents in a chronic phase (defined in this classification as Stage I) which may be associated with symptoms such as abdominal fullness due to splenomegaly. Alternately, many cases of CML are initially asymptomatic and are detected by a complete blood count performed for unrelated reasons. The chronic phase has a quite variable duration lasting from months to many years with a median duration of 3–4 years. The chronic phase evolves through an accelerated phase (defined as Stage II) characterized by increasing immaturity of the white blood cells in the blood or marrow. Since the accelerated phase is invariably followed by the life-threatening acute phase (defined as Stage III) more drastic therapeutic measures are instituted at this point. Death from CML is usually due to blastic infiltration and haemorrhage or infection in Stage III.

Until recently, treatment during the chronic phase employed chemotherapy aimed primarily at controlling the symptoms resulting from an enlarged spleen or very high leucocyte or platelet count. There was little evidence that treatment during the chronic phase affected the progression of CML or overall survival. However, current therapies for CML in addition to chemotherapy include bone marrow transplantation and biological therapies such as interferon. Bone marrow transplantation offers a clear opportunity at cure of this disease. Interferon therapy may slow the progression of the disease in some patients. The treatment of accelerated phase or acute phase (also called blast crisis) is handled similarly to the treatment of any acute leukaemia in an adult. Overall the acute phase of CML is even more refractory to treatment than acute leukaemia arising de novo.

Rationale for Staging

The purpose of a staging system is to recognize the life history of a tumour and to apply that knowledge to a particular patient. CML is recognized to have three distinct clinical phases. To study this disease and the effects of new therapies, it is necessary that these phases be accurately described in a staging system. Physicians wishing to provide new therapies for their patients must know how to compare them to the results described in clinical trials. The proposed staging system for monitoring of CML patients defines three stages in a manner which conforms with clinical studies of the progression of this disease. Similar to the standard anatomically based TNM staging of cancer, the CML staging system uses three factors as indices which are then combined into a single stage.

References and Bibliography for CML

Ayscue LH, Ross DW, Ozer H, Rao K, Gulley ML, Dent GA (1990) Bcr/abl recombinant DNA analysis versus karyotype in the diagnosis and therapeutic monitoring of chronic myeloid leukemia. Am J Clin Pathol 94: 404–409

Arlin ZA, Silver RT, Bennett JM (1990) Blastic phase of chronic myeloid leukemia (blCML): a proposal for standardization of diagnostic and response criteria. Leukemia 11: 755–757

Cervantes F, Rozman C (1982) A multivariate analysis of prognostic factors in chronic myeloid leukemia. Blood 60: 1298–1304

Cervantes F, Rozman M, Rosell J et al (1990) A study of prognostic factors in blast crisis of Philadelphia chromosome-positive chronic myelogenous leukemia. Br J Haematol 76: 27–32

Kantarjian HM, Keating MJ, Talpaz M, et al (1987) Chronic myelogenous leukemia in blast crisis. Am J Med 83: 445–454

Kantarjian HM, Dixon D, Keating MJ, et al (1988) Characteristics of accelerated disease in chronic myelogenous leukemia. Cancer 61: 1441–1446

Muehleck SD, McKenna RW, Arthur DC, et al (1984) Transformation of chronic myelogenous leukemia: clinical morphologic, and cytogenetic features. AJCP July: 1–14

Ross DN, Brunning RD, Kantarjian HM, Koeffler HP, Ozer H (1993) A proposed staging system for chronic myeloid leukemia. Cancer 71: 3788–3791

Sokal JE, Cox EB, Baccarani M, et al (1984) Prognostic discrimination in "good-risk" chronic granulocytic leukemia. Blood 63: 789–799

Swolin B, Weinfeld A, Westin J, et al (1985) Karyotypic evolution in Ph-positive chronic myeloid leukemia in relation to management and disease progression. Cancer Genet Cytogenet 18: 65–79

Terjanian T, Kantarjian H, Keating M, et al (1987) Clinical and prognostic features of patients with Philadelphia chromosome-positive chronic myelogenous leukemia and extramedullary disease. Cancer 59: 297–300

Tura S, Baccarani M, Corbelli G, and the Italian Cooperative Study Group on Chronic Myeloid Leukemia (1981) Staging of chronic myeloid leukemia. Br J Haematol 47: 105–119

Primary Liver Carcinoma in Infants and Children

The following classification has been proposed by the Japanese TNM Committee. It is based on the examination in 136 cases of hepatoblastoma seen in 14 Japanese institutions (Morita et al. 1983).

Rules for Classification

The classification applies to primary liver carcinoma in patients age 16 years or less. In this age predominantly hepatoblastoma is observed, while hepatocellular carcinoma is uncommon. There should be histological verification of the disease.

The following are the procedures for assessment of the T, N and M categories:

T categories   Physical examination, imaging and/or surgical exploration
N categories   Physical examination, imaging and/or surgical exploration
M categories   Physical examination, imaging and/or surgical exploration

Regional Lymph Nodes

The regional lymph nodes are the suprahepatic, infrahepatic, hilar, hepatoduodenal, pancreaticoduodenal and coeliac nodes.

TNM Clinical Classification

T – Primary Tumour

TX   Primary tumour cannot be assessed
T0   No evidence of primary tumour

T1   Tumour confined to one segment of the liver
T2   Tumour confined to two segments of the liver
T3   Tumour confined to three segments of the liver
T4   Tumour involving more than three segments of the liver

Note. For staging purposes the liver is subdivided into 8 segments (Couinaud 1957).

N – Regional Lymph Nodes

NX   Regional lymph nodes cannot be assessed
N0   No regional lymph node metastasis
N1   Metastasis to suprahepatic, infrahepatic, hilar or hepatoduodenal lymph nodes
N2   Metastasis to pancreaticoduodenal or coeliac lymph nodes

M – Distant Metastasis

MX   Presence of distant metastasis cannot be assessed
M0   No distant metastasis
M1   Distant metastasis

pTNM Pathological Classification

The pT, pN and pM categories correspond to the T, N and M categories.

Stage Grouping

Stage I	T1	N0	M0
Stage II	T2	N0	M0
Stage IIIA	T3	N0	M0
Stage IIIB	T1	N1, 2	M0
	T2	N1, 2	M0
	T3	N1, 2	M0
	T4	Any N	M0
Stage IV	Any T	Any N	M1

Summary

Primary Liver Carcinoma in Infants and Children	
T1	One segment
T2	2 segments
T3	3 segments
T4	> 3 segments
N1	Suprahepatic, infrahepatic, hilar, hepatoduodenal
N2	Pancreaticoduodenal, coeliac

References

Bunn PA, Lamberg SI (1979) Report of the committee on staging and classification of cutaneous T-cell lymphomas. Cancer Treatment Rep 63: 725–728

Burg G, Sterry W, EORTC/BMFT Cutaneous Lymphoma Project Group (1987) Recommendations for staging and therapy of cutaneous lymphomas. A European concept. EORTC/BMFT, Würzburg

Calearo C (1990) Annual Report of ICC to UICC. Unpublished internal manuscript

Couinaud C (1957) Le Foie. Etudes Anatomiques et chirurgicales. Masson, Paris

Creasman WT (1992) Revision in classification by the International Federation of Gynecology and Obstetrics. Am J Obstet Gynecol 167: 857–858

International League of Dermatological Societies, Committee on Nomenclature (1987) Glossary of basic dermatology lesions. Almquist and Wiksell, Uppsala

Morita K, Okabe I, Uchino J, Watanabe I, Iwabuchi M, Matsuyama S, Takahashi H, Nakajo T, Hirai Y, Tsuchida Y, Katsumata K, Hasegawa H, Nishi T, Okamoto E, Ikeda K (1983) The proposed Japanese TNM classification of primary liver carcinoma in infants and children. Jpn J Clin Oncol 13: 361–370

Rosai J, Levine GD (1976) Tumors of the thymus. AFIP, Washington, DC

Schwab W (1990) Personal communication

Schwab W, Clasen B, Steinhoff HJ (1988) Erfahrungsbericht (1974–1986) zur Klassifizierung und Lokalisationsverteilung von malignen Tumoren des Organs Innere Nase und Nebenhöhlen. HNO 36: 154–157

Yamakawa Y, Masaoka A, Hashimoto T, Niwa H, Muzino T, Fujii Y, Nakahara K (1991) A tentative tumor-node-metastasis classification of thymoma. Cancer 68: 1984–1987

Optional Proposals for Testing New Telescopic Ramifications of TNM

Introduction

In this chapter, various proposals for optional subdivision of the existing T, N and M categories, i.e. "telescopic" ramification, are presented. Telescoping accomodates the collection of additional data without altering the definitions of the existing TNM categories.

The concept of telescoping permits an orderly expansion of TNM elements to allow for (1) testing of subcategories for prognosis and (2) treatment planning considerations. Telescoping accomodates "splitters" and "lumpers", permits data from expansions to collapse into the standard categories and promotes testing of new hypotheses uniformly in different centres.

The editors recognize that staging has to be simple enough for universal use in both highly developed and developing countries and sufficiently uncomplicated so that medical professionals are not discouraged from using the system. On the other side, for specialized institutions and for investigational purposes a relatively simple staging system is not sufficient and runs the risk of not being used. For these specialized institutions the TNM system may be made attractive by further subdivision of the existing categories (telescopic ramification) and by including additional descriptors.

The proposals for subdivisions and additional designations in this section are presented for investigational use and are *entirely optional*. Some proposals relate to subclassifications of M1 and are of interest to medical oncologists. Justification for each proposal is given based on published data or clinical experience.

All Tumour Sites

Fixation of Lymph Nodes

Some clinicians believe that fixation of nodes is important for treatment planning. For analysis, fixation may be specified within the existing N categories e.g. N1, N2 or N3.

Micrometastasis

pN 1   Cases with micrometastasis only, i. e. no metastasis larger than 0.2 cm, can be identified by the addition of "(mi)", e. g. pN 1(mi) or pN 2(mi).

In breast cancer this does not apply because size of metastasis is already considered in the pN classification.

Justification. Historical considerations, general experience.

pM 1   Micrometastasis, i. e. no metastasis larger than 0.2 cm, in viscera (lung, liver, etc.) or bone marrow can be identified by the addition of "(mi)", e. g. M 1(mi).

Isolated tumour cells found in bone marrow may be indicated by the addition of "(i)", e. g. M 1(i).

Justification. The clinical and prognostic significance of finding isolated tumour cells is as yet unproven. Selected literature on detection and prognostic significance of occult tumour cells in the bone marrow: Mansi et al. (1987, 1989), Ceci et al. (1988), Cote et al. (1988, 1991), Kirk et al. (1990), Salvadori et al. (1990), Schlimok et al. (1990, 1991, 1992), Molino et al. (1991), Jauch et al. (1992), Lindemann et al. (1992).

Markers of Residual Tumour

R0   R0a   Negative markers after tumour resection for cure (R0)
      R0b   Persistently elevated marker level or rising marker level within 4 months after tumour resection for cure
             Justification. General considerations, general experience.

Head and Neck Tumours

N Classification Proposal 1
Larynx Carcinoma

Based on data on surgically treated patients with larynx carcinoma the following proposal for the N classification was presented by Glanz (1992). It is a slight modification of an earlier proposal published in 1989 by Glanz and Eichhorn.

Proposed N Classification of Glanz (1992)

N0   No regional lymph node metastasis
N1   Metastasis in one or two unilateral regional lymph nodes of the upper two thirds of neck,[1] not more than 2 cm in greatest dimension, without extension beyond lymph node capsule

N2   Regional lymph node metastasis in the upper two thirds of neck without extension beyond lymph node capsule if
    – bilateral, or
    – more than two nodes involved, or
    – more than 2 cm in greatest dimension
N3   Regional lymph node metastasis, any with extension beyond lymph node capsule[2] *or* any in the lower third of neck

Notes
1. The border between the upper two and the lower third is the plane of the intermediate tendon over the jugular vein dividing the omohyoid muscle into two bellies.
2. For clinical classification, extension beyond the lymph node capsule corresponds to involved node(s) fixed to one another or to other structures.

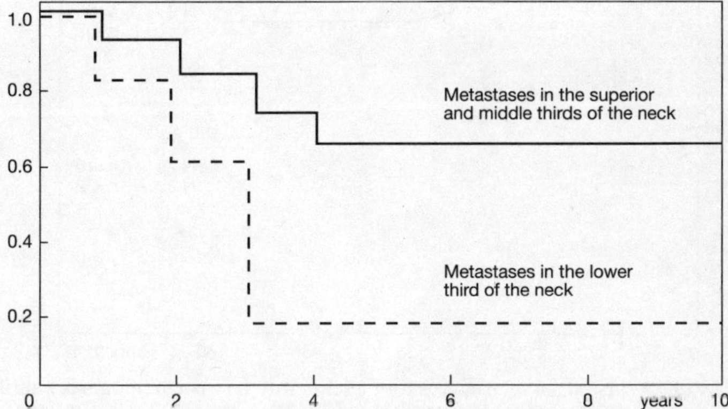

Fig. 17. Larynx carcinoma. Prognosis after surgical treatment including neck dissection. Patients with histologically proven regional lymph node metastasis. Adjusted survival in relation to the site of lymph node metastasis. For definition of levels see text. (From Glanz and Eichhorn 1989)

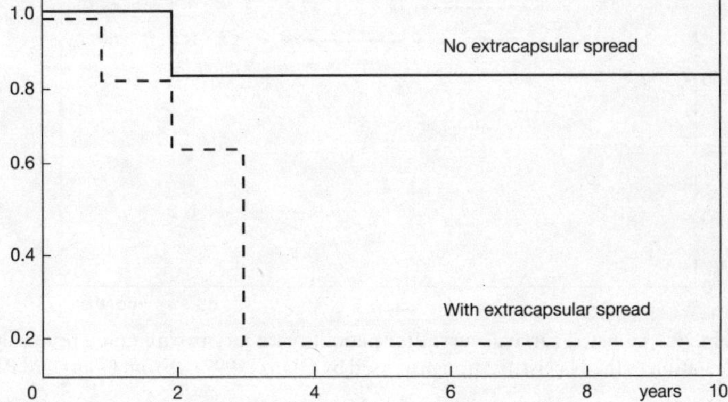

Fig. 18. Larynx carcinoma. Prognosis after surgical treatment including neck dissection. Patients with histologically proven regional lymph node metastasis. Adjusted survival in relation to extracapsular spread. (From Glanz and Eichhorn 1989)

Justification. The UICC N classification considers number, site and size of metastasis. The categories for number are single/multiple, for site ipsilateral/bi- or contralateral, for size ≤ 3 cm/$> 3–6$ cm/> 6 cm. According to Glanz and Eichhorn (1989), other boundaries are preferable with regard to prognostic significance, namely for number $1–2/> 2$ and for size ≤ 2 cm/> 2 cm. Furthermore, a significant influence of the level of metastasis (upper two thirds versus lower third) (Fig. 17) and of perinodular spread of metastasis (Fig. 18) was demonstrated.

Figures 19 and 20 show the survival of larynx carcinoma patients in relation to the present UICC N classification and to the classification proposed by Glanz (1992).

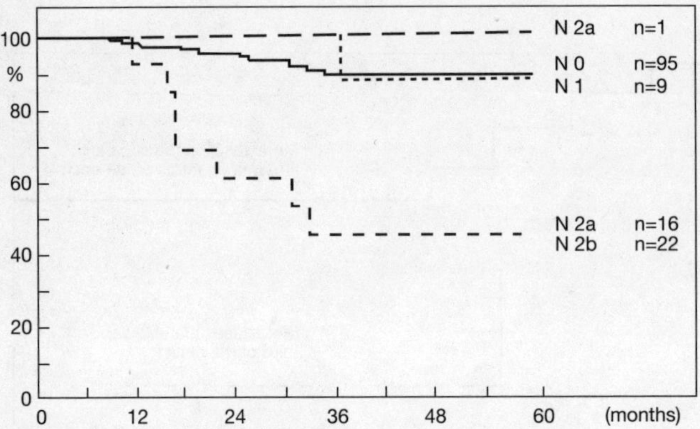

Fig. 19. Adjusted survival curves for patients with larynx carcinoma primarily treated surgically. Relation to the UICC N classification of 1987. (From Glanz and Popella 1993)

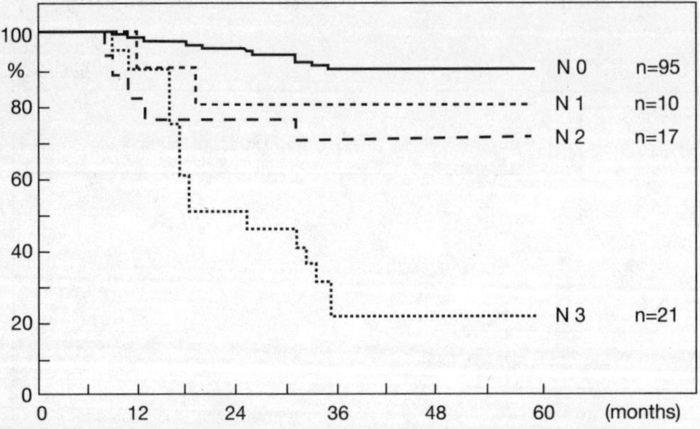

Fig. 20. Adjusted survival curves for patients with larynx carcinoma primarily treated surgically. Relation to the N classification proposed by Glanz (1992). (From Glanz and Popella 1993)

**Ramification of Present N Classification
(Any Site Except Thyroid and Nasopharynx)**

The following ramification of the present UICC classification will enable a future comparison between the present UICC classification and the classification of Glanz (1992). Because the latter is based on data from larynx carcinoma patients, not only must its superiority for larynx be investigated but also whether it can be used for patients with carcinomas of other head and neck sites (except thyroid).

N 1 (unilateral, single, $\leq$ 3 cm)	(i) metastasis in upper two thirds, 2 cm or less in greatest dimension, no extension beyond capsule
	(ii) Metastasis in upper two thirds, more than 2 cm but not more than 3 cm in greatest dimension, no extension beyond capsule
	(iii) Metastasis in lower third *or* extension beyond capsule
N 2 a (ipsilateral, single, > 3–6 cm)	(i) Metastasis in upper two thirds, no extension beyond capsule
	(ii) Metastasis in lower third *or* extension beyond capsule
N 2 b (ipsilateral, multiple, $\leqslant$ 6 cm)	(i) Metastasis in two nodes in upper two thirds, 2 cm or less in greatest dimension, no extension beyond capsule
	(ii) Metastasis in more than 2 nodes in upper two thirds, 2 cm or less in greatest dimension, no extension beyond capsule
	(iii) Metastasis in upper two thirds, more than 2 cm but not more than 6 cm in greatest dimension, no extension beyond capsule
	(iv) Metastasis in lower third *or* extension beyond capsule
N 2 c (bilateral, contralateral, $\leqslant$ 6 cm)	(i) Metastasis in upper two thirds, no extension beyond capsule
	(ii) Metastasis in lower third *or* extension beyond capsule
N 3 (> 6 cm)	(i) Metastasis in upper two thirds, no extension beyond capsule
	(ii) Metastasis in lower third *or* extension beyond capsule

Conversion Tables

UICC	Glanz (1992)		Glanz (1992)	UICC
N1(i)	N1		N1	N1(i)
N1(ii)	N2			N2b(i)
N1(iii)	N3		N2	N1(ii)
N2a(i)	N2			N2a(i)
N2a(ii)	N3			N2b(ii)
N2b(i)	N1			N2b(iii)
N2b(ii)	N2			N2c(i)
N2b(iii)	N2			N3(i)
N2b(iv)	N3		N3	N1(iii)
N2c(i)	N2			N2a(ii)
N2c(ii)	N3			N2b(iv)
N3(i)	N2			N2c(ii)
N3(ii)	N3			N3(ii)

N Classification Proposal 2
Any Site Except Thyroid and Nasopharynx

N3   N3a   Metastasis in a single ipsilateral lymph node more than 6 cm in
              greatest dimension

     N3b   Metastasis in multiple ipsilateral lymph nodes, at least one more
              than 6 cm in greatest dimension

     N3c   Metastasis in bilateral or contralateral lymph nodes, at least one
              more than 6 cm in greatest dimension

Justification. Further clarification of prognosis for the various subgroups needed
(DSK-TNM)

Lip and Oral Cavity

Various observations from different groups (see Platz et al. 1986) indicated that tumour thickness measured in millimeters is of great influence on patients' prognosis. Therefore, the German–Austrian–Swiss Working Group on Tumours in the Maxillofacial Region (DÖSAK) (Hausamen 1988) analysed the material in its tumour registry (Howaldt et al. 1991) and elaborated a new T classification considering greatest horizontal dimension of tumour as well as tumour thickness. The latter was assessed by clinical examination and, if feasible, also by CT scan.

Proposed T Classification of Howaldt et al. (1992)

T1   Tumour 2 cm or less in greatest dimension and 5 mm or less in thickness
T2   Tumour 2 cm or less in greatest dimension and more than 5 mm but not more
than 10 mm in thickness *or*
tumour more than 2 cm but not more than 4 cm in greatest dimension and
5 mm or less in thickness
T3   Tumour 2 cm or less in greatest dimension and more than 10 mm but not
more than 20 mm in thickness *or*
tumour more than 2 cm but not more than 4 cm in greatest dimension and
more than 5 mm but not more than 20 mm in thickness *or*
tumour more than 4 cm in thickness and 5 mm or less in thickness
T4   Tumour more than 4 cm in greatest dimension and more than 5 mm in thickness *or*
tumour of any size and more than 20 mm in thickness
    T4a   Tumour more than 4 cm in greatest dimension and more than 5 mm
but not more than 20 mm in thickness
    T4b   Tumour 4 cm or less in greatest dimension and more than 20 mm in
thickness
    T4c   Tumour more than 4 cm in greatest dimension and more than 20 mm
in thickness

Summary

Greatest dimension (horizontal)	Tumour thickness			
	≤ 5 mm	> 5–10 mm	> 10–20 mm	> 20 mm
≤ 20 mm	T1	T2	T3	T4b
> 20–40 mm	T2	T3	T3	T4b
> 40 mm	T3	T4a	T4a	T4c

Justification. The proposed classification is based on follow-up data from 2786 patients with squamous cell carcinoma of the lip and oral cavity. Figures 21 and 22 show the survival in relation to the present TNM classification and to the proposed new classification. The better discrimination is clearly demonstrated.

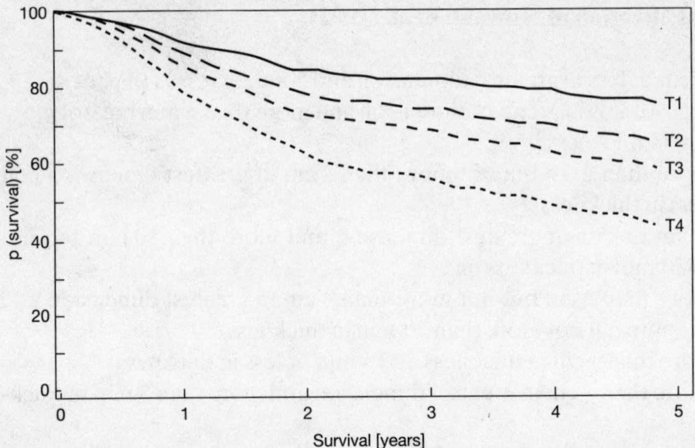

Fig. 21. Observed survival in relation to the present UICC T classification. Squamous cell carcinoma of lip and oral cavity, NOMO: T1, $n = 622$; T2, $n = 757$; T3, $n = 184$; T4, $n = 1223$. (From Howaldt et al. 1992)

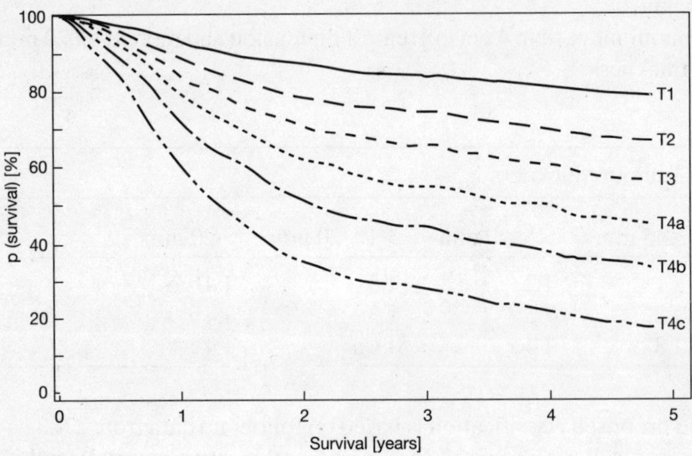

Fig. 22. Observed survival in relation to the proposed T classification. Same patients as in Fig. 21. T1; $n = 516$; T2, $n = 630$; T3, $n = 985$, T4a, $n = 444$; T4b, $n = 48$, T4c, $n = 163$. (From Howaldt et al. 1992)

Ramification of Present T Classification

To enable a comparison between the present UICC and the proposed T classification, the following ramification of the UICC classification is proposed.

T1, T2, T3   (i)   5 mm or less in thickness
                 (ii) More than 5 mm but not more than 10 mm in thickness
                 (iii) More than 10 mm but not more than 20 mm in thickness
                 (iv) More than 20 mm in thickness

T4   (i)   20 mm or less in greatest dimension and 5 mm
                  or less in thickness

           (ii)   20 mm or less in greatest dimension and more than
                  5 mm but not more than 10 mm in thickness *or*
                  More than 20 mm but not more than 40 mm in
                  greatest dimension and 5 mm or less in thickness

          (iii)   20 mm or less in greatest dimension and more than
                  10 mm but not more than 20 mm in thickness *or*
                  More than 20 mm but not more than 40 mm in
                  greatest dimension and more than 5 mm but not
                  more than 20 mm in thickness *or*
                  More than 40 mm in greatest dimension and 5 mm
                  or less in thickness

          (iv)   More than 40 mm in greatest dimension and more than
                  5 mm but not more than 20 mm in thickness

           (v)   40 mm or less in greatest dimension and more than
                  20 mm in thickness

          (vi)   More than 40 mm in greatest dimension and more
                  than 20 mm in thickness

Conversion Tables

UICC	Howaldt et al. (1992)
T1(i)	T1
T1(ii)	T2
T1(iii)	T3
T1(iv)	T4b
T2(i)	T2
T2(ii)	T3
T2(iii)	T3
T2(iv)	T4b
T3(i)	T3
T3(ii)	T4a
T3(iii)	T4a
T3(iv)	T4c
T4(i)	T1
T4(ii)	T2
T4(iii)	T3
T4(iv)	T4a
T4(v)	T4b
T4(vi)	T4c

Howaldt et al. (1992)	UICC
T1	T1(i)
	T4(i)
T2	T1(ii)
	T2(i)
	T4(ii)
T3	T1(iii)
	T2(ii)
	T2(iii)
	T3(i)
	T4(iii)
T4a	T3(ii)
	T3(iii)
	T4(iv)
T4b	T1(iv)
	T2(iv)
	T4(v)
T4c	T3(iv)
	T4(vi)

Hypopharynx

T Classification

T1   T1a   2 cm or less
     T1b   More than 2 cm but not more than 4 cm
     T1c   More than 4 cm

Justification. Treatment planning (DSK-TNM 1991).

Nasopharynx

Nasopharynx carcinoma has a peculiar geographic distribution with a high incidence in southeastern Asia. In this area the staging system of Ho (1970, 1978 a, b) is frequently used.

Staging System of Ho

T – Primary Tumour

T1   Tumour confined to the nasopharynx (space behind the choanal orifices and nasal septum and above the posterior margin of the soft palate in the resting position)

T2   Tumour extended to the nasal fossa, oropharynx or adjacent muscles or nerves below the base of the skull

T3   Tumour extending beyond T2 limits and subclassified as follows:

     T3a   Bone involvement below the base of the skull (including floor of sphenoid sinus)

     T3b   Involvement of base of skull

     T3c   Involvement of cranial nerve(s) at or above the base of skull (cranial extension)

     T3d   Involvement of orbit, laryngopharynx (hypopharynx) or infratemporal fossa

N – Regional Lymph Nodes

N0   No palpable nodes

N1   Palpable node(s) wholly in upper cervical level, bounded below by the neck crease extending laterally and backwards from or just below the thyroid notch (laryngeal eminence)

N2   Palpable node(s) between the crease and the supraclavicular fossa, the upper limit being a line joining the upper margin of the sternal end of the clavicle and the apex of an angle formed by the lateral surface of the neck and the superior margin of the trapezius

N3   Palpable node(s) in the supraclavicular fossa and/or skin involvement in the form of carcinoma en cuirasse or satellite nodules above the clavicles

Ramification of Present T and N classifications

To enable comparison between staging according to Ho and the present UICC staging system the following ramifications of the UICC system are proposed.

T Classification

T4   T4a   Invasion of any of the last 4 cranial nerves below the base of the skull

T4b   Bone involvement below the base of the skull (including the floor but not the roof or lateral walls of the sphenoid sinus, pterygoid lamina, nasal septum, bony wall(s) of the maxillary of ethmoidal sinus and/or cervical spine by direct invasion)

T4c   Involvement of base of skull

T4d   Involvement of cranial nerve(s) at or above the base of skull

T4e   Involvement of orbit, laryngopharynx (hypopharynx) or infratemporal fossa

Note: Involvement of any of the last 4 cranial nerves within the retrostyloid parapharyngeal space is considered to be involvement of the base of the skull (T4c) because the jugular foramen forms a part of the upper border of the space and it is highly probable that there is already perineural spread higher up by the time the nerve(s) show clinical involvement.

N Classification

Any of the present N categories may be subdivided into:

(i)   Limited to upper cervical level
(ii)   Involvement of lower cervical level
(iii)   Involvement of supraclavicular level
(iv)   Involvement of supraclavicular level and skin

Note. The levels are defined as follows:
- Upper cervical: above the neck crease that extends laterally and backwards from or just below the thyroid notch (laryngeal eminence)
- Lower cervical: between the neck crease (see above) and a line joining the upper margin of the sternal end of the clavicle and the apex of an angle formed by the lateral surface of the neck and the superior margin of the trapezius
- Supraclavicular: below the line defined as the lower border of the lower cervical level (see above), that is, in the supraclavicular fossa.

Conversion Tables

UICC	Ho
T1	T1
T2	T1
T3	T2
T4a	T2
T4b	T3a
T4c	T3b
T4d	T3c
T4e	T3d
N0	N0
N1(i)	N1
N1(ii)	N2
N1(iii)	N3
N1(iv)	N3
N2(i)	N1
N2(ii)	N2
N2(iii)	N3
N2(iv)	N3
N3(i)	N1
N3(ii)	N2
N3(iii)	N3
N3(iv)	N3

Ho	UICC
T1	T1
	T2
T2	T3
	T4a
T3a	T4b
T3b	T4c
T3c	T4d
T3d	T4e
N0	N0
N1	N1(i)
	N2(i)
	N3(i)
N2	N1(ii)
	N2(ii)
	N3(ii)
N3	N1(iii)
	N1(iv)
	N2(iii)
	N2(iv)
	N3(iii)
	N3(iv)

Note. Comparison of the classifications applied to the same patients may show the value of each of their components and provide justification for future revisions.

Invasive Larynx Carcinoma

The T and pT classifications of invasive larynx carcinoma have been criticized and discussed during recent years (Glanz 1984, 1986; Kleinsasser 1986, 1992; Alajmo et al. 1988; Karim et al. 1990; Meyer-Breiting 1990; Molinari 1990; Bittesini et al. 1991; Calearo 1991; Meyer-Breiting and Bettinger 1991; Popella et al. 1991; Wolfensberger 1992). In the following, a T classification is presented which is based primarily on the proposals of Glanz (1984, 1986) and Kleinsasser (1986, 1992) and considers modifications proposed to the German Head and Neck Society for all head and neck tumours by Steiner and Ambrosch (1993) as a basis for further ramification studies.

T and pT Classification: Modified Proposal of Kleinsasser and Glanz

The classification applies to supraglottis, glottis and subglottis.

T1   Tumour 15 mm or less in greatest dimension, with normal vocal cord mobility

T2   Tumor more than 15 mm in greatest dimension, with normal vocal cord motility

    T2a   Tumour more than 15 mm but not more than 25 mm in greatest dimension, with normal vocal cord mobility

    T2b   Tumour more than 25 mm in greatest dimension, with normal vocal cord mobility

T3   Tumour with impaired vocal cord mobility or vocal cord fixation, limited to the larynx

T4   Tumour extends beyond larynx to adjacent structures

Notes

1. Vocal cord mobility is a criterion for the T classification only in tumours of the glottis.
2. Greatest dimension relates to horizontal spread.
3. For classification of bilateral tumours, the extension on both sides is added together.
4. T2b corresponds to the so-called superficial spreading carcinoma.
5. In tumours of the supraglottis, invasion of the postcricoid area, medial wall of piriform sinus or pre-epiglottic tissues is classified T3.
6. Carcinoma of the glottis may be further divided into (I) (unilateral) and (II) bilateral
7. A superficical extension, i.e. extension limited to the mucosa, beyond the larynx does not qualify for T4 (see p.21).
8. The outer borders of the larynx are the outer perichondrium of the thyroid cartilage, the hyothyroid and cricothyroid membrane, the lower margin of the cricoid cartilage, the margins of the aryepiglottic folds and the arytenoid region.
9. The pT categories correspond to the T categories. For classification, histological tumour invasion of more than 5 mm corresponds to impaired vocal cord mobility or vocal cord fixation.

Justification. This classification has the following advantages:

– Uniform classification for each site of larynx.
– Classification by greatest dimension is used in the TNM classification for many sites and is more reproducible than classification by subsites, which are only partly defined.
– The assessment of the greatest dimension is possible during indirect or direct laryngoscopy.
– The proposed T categories are more homogeneous with regard to prognosis, especially in the T2 category.
– The classification has a direct bearing on treatment, especially T2 versus T3.

Figure 23 shows the adjusted survival in relation to the T categories of Kleinsasser (1992)

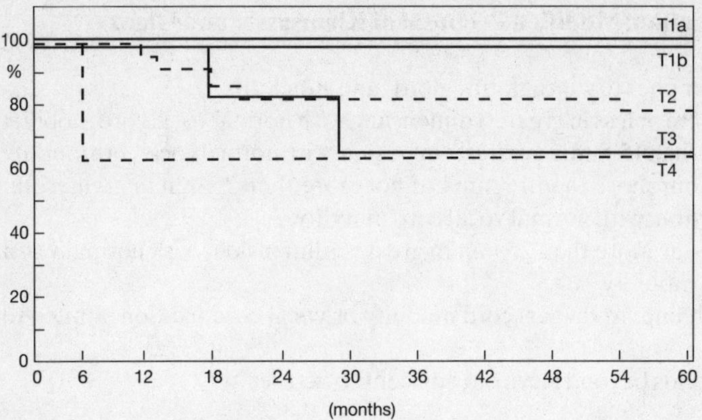

Fig. 23. Adjusted survival curves for glottis carcinoma treated primarily by surgery (any N, M0): prognosis in relation to the proposed T categories. T1a, $n = 125$; T1b, $n = 22$; T2, $n = 45$; T3, $n = 28$; T4, $n = 4$. (From Kleinsasser 1992)

In surgically treated patients the additional consideration of depth of invasion improves prediction of prognosis. The better discrimination of survival by pT is seen on comparison of Figs. 23 and 24.

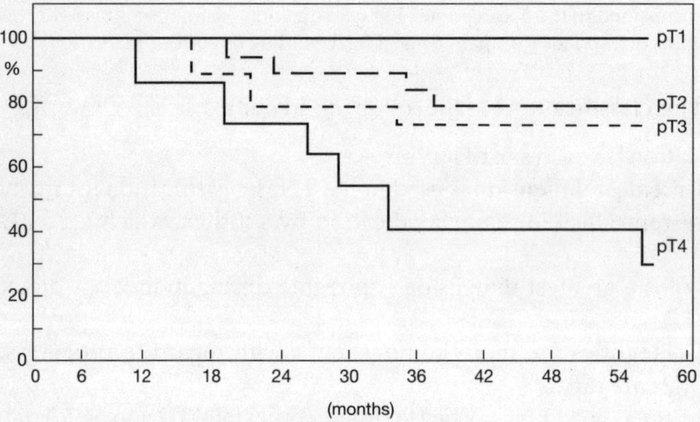

Fig. 24. Adjusted survival curves for glottis carcinoma treated primarily by surgery (any N, M0): prognosis in relation to the proposed pT classification. pT1, $n = 124$; pT2, $n = 57$; pT3, $n = 26$; pT4, $n = 17$. (From Kleinsasser 1992)

Ramification of Present T Classification

To enable comparisons between the modified proposal of Kleinsasser and Glanz for the T classification (see p. 113) and the present UICC classification, the following ramification of the UICC system is proposed.

Supraglottis
   T1, T2   (i) $\leqslant$ 15 mm
                (ii) > 15–25 mm
                (iii) > 25 mm

Glottis
   T1a, T1b   (i) $\leqslant$ 15 mm
                (ii) > 15–25 mm
                (iii) > 25 mm
   T2   (i)   Normal vocal cord mobility, $\leq$ 15 mm
                (ii) Normal vocal cord mobility, > 15–25 mm
                (iii) Normal vocal cord mobility, > 25 mm
                (iv) Impaired vocal cord mobility

Subglottis
   T1   As T1a and T1b in glottis
   T2   As in glottis

By using this ramification it is possible to classify each case according to the UICC system as well as according to the modified proposal of Kleinsasser and Glanz (see p. 113). Comparison of the respective survival curves and rates may indicate which classification is superior.

Conversion Tables

	UICC	Kleinsasser and Glanz	Kleinsasser and Glanz	UICC
Supraglottis	T1(i)	T1	T1	T1(i)
	T1(ii)	T2a		T2(i)
	T1(iii)	T2b	T2a	T1(ii)
	T2(i)	T1		T2(ii)
	T2(ii)	T2a	T2b	T1(iii)
	T2(iii)	T2b		T2(iii)
	T3	T3	T3	T3
	T4	T4	T4	T4
Glottis	T1a(i)	T1(i)	T1(i)	T1a(i)
	T1a(ii)	T2a(i)		T2(i)
	T1a(iii)	T2b(i)	T1(ii)	T1b(i)
	T1b(i)	T1(ii)		T2(i)
	T1b(ii)	T2a(ii)	T2a(i)	T1a(i)
	T1b(iii)	T2b(ii)		T2(ii)
	T2(i)	T1(i)	T2a(ii)	T1b(ii)
		T1(ii)		T2(ii)
	T2(ii)	T2a(i)	T2b(i)	T1a(iii)
		T2a(ii)		T2(iii)
	T2(iii)	T2b(i)	T2b(ii)	T1b(iii)
		T2b(ii)		T2(iii)
	T2(iv)	T3	T3	T2(iv)
	T3	T3		T3
	T4	T4	T4	T4
Subglottis	T1(i)	T1	T1	T1(i)
	T1(ii)	T2a		T2(i)
	T1(iii)	T2b	T2a	T1(ii)
	T2(i)	T1		T2a(ii)
	T2(ii)	T2a	T2b	T1(iii)
	T2(iii)	T2b		T2(iii)
	T2(iv)	T3	T3	T2(iv)
	T3	T3		T3
	T4	T4	T4	T4

It should be emphasized that Kleinsasser and Glanz propose dropping the differentiation between glottis and subglottis (see Fleischer 1977; Glanz 1984; Kleinsasser 1992).

Noninvasive Larynx Carcinoma

T Classification

Tis (i) 15 mm or less in greatest dimension
     (ii) More than 15 mm in greatest dimension

Note. In bilateral tumours the greatest dimensions of tumours on both sides are added up for classification.

Justification. Glanz and Popella (1993) demonstrated the worse prognosis in Tis(ii) (Fig. 25).

Maxillary Sinus

Proposed T Classification of Steiner and Ambrosch (1992)

T1   Tumour limited to mucosa of the site with no erosion or destruction of bone
T2   Tumour with superficial extension into adjacent site(s) or with erosion of bone
      T2a   Tumour with superficial extension to adjacent site(s)
      T2b   Tumour with erosion of bone
T3   Tumour with destruction of bone
T4   Tumour with invasion through bone into adjacent structures

Note. *Erosion* of bone is invasion of cortex only, *destruction* is invasion into spongiosa.

At present, supporting data are not available. It is possible that the classification could also be used for other paranasal sinuses.

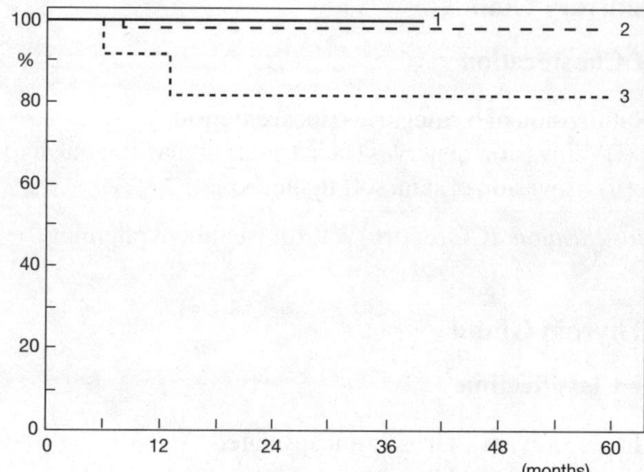

Fig. 25. Carcinoma in situ of the glottis treated by endolaryngeal surgery: adjusted survival curves. *1,* pTis(i), unilateral, $n = 4$; *2,* pTis(i), bilateral, $n = 60$; *3;* pTis(ii), $n = 12$. (From Glanz and Popella 1993)

Ramification of Present T Classification

To enable a future comparison of the present UICC classification and the classification of Steiner and Ambrosch (1992) the following ramification of the UICC classification is proposed:

T1	T1a	Limited to the site
	T1b	With superficial extension to adjacent site(s)
T2	T2a	With erosion of bone
	T2b	With destruction of bone
T3	T3a	With invasion of posterior wall of the maxillary sinus, floor or medial wall of orbit
	T3b	With invasion through bone to cheek or anterior ethmoid sinus

Conversion Tables

UICC ramified	Steiner and Ambrosch (1992)	Steiner and Ambrosch (1992)	UICC ramified
T1a	T1	T1	T1a
T1b	T2a	T2a	T1b
T2a	T2b	T2b	T2a
T2b	T3	T3	T2b
T3a	T3		T3b
T3b	T4	T4	T3b
T4	T4		T4

Justification. ICC report of 1992 indicates that the present UICC classification ist too complex.

Salivary Glands

T Classification

Subdivision of b categories (local extension):
b(i)   Invasion of nerves (facial, mandibular, lingual, hypoglossal)
b(ii) Invasion of skin, soft tissue, bone

Justification. ICC report 1989, for treatment planning.

Thyroid Gland

T Classification

T1, 2, 3 a,b   (i) Grossly encapsulated
               (ii) Grossly nonencapsulated

Justification. Different prognosis and treatment, especially for follicular carcinoma in patients under 45 years (ECC).

N Classification

N 1 a   (i)   Metastasis in ipsilateral central cervical lymph nodes
         (ii)   Metastasis in ipsilateral lateral cervical lymph nodes
N 1 b   (i)   Metastasis in bilateral or contralateral central or midline cervical
                lymph nodes
         (ii)   Metastasis in bilateral or contralateral lateral cervical lymph nodes
         (iii) Metastasis in mediastinal lymph nodes

Note. The *central* cervical lymph nodes are the submandibular, submental, prelaryngeal and paratracheal (supra-, peri-, infrathyroidal, pretracheal) lymph nodes.
The *lateral* cervical lymph nodes are the superficial and deep lateral cervical and the supraclavicular nodes (see p. 22 ff).

Justification. Treatment planning (Dralle 1992; Dralle et al. 1993).

Digestive System Tumours

All Sites Except Oesophagus

M Classification

M 1   M 1 a   Metastasis in nonregional lymph nodes only
       M 1 b   Metastasis in viscera (excluding peritoneal and pleural metastasis)
       M 1 c   Peritoneal and pleural metastasis

Justification. Different prognosis, response to chemotherapy, and treatment (ECC).

Oesophagus

T Classification

T 1   T 1 a   Tumour invades lamina propria
       T 1 b   Tumour invades submucosa

Justification. Different frequency of lymph node metastasis, different prognosis, important indication for treatment by laser and limited endoscopic procedures (Endo et al. 1988; Hirayama and Mori 1990; Yoshinaka et al. 1991; Tajiri 1992)

N Classification

N1   N1a   1–3 nodes involved
       N1b   4–7 nodes involved
       N1c   > 7 nodes involved

Justification. Different prognosis in relation to the number of involved lymph nodes demonstrated by Siewert 1992: Squamous cell carcinoma of the intra-thoracic oesophagus treated by surgical resection (any R), surgical mortality not excluded (Kaplan–Meier):

	Number of patients	2-year survival rate (%)	5-year survival rate (%)	Median survival time (months)
pN1a	58	22	11	12
pN1b	32	18	0	9
pN1c	19	0	0	6

The difference was statistically significant ($p < 0.05$).

The importance of the number of involved lymph nodes has been confirmed recently by Kato et al. (1993), Matsubara et al. (1993) and Roder et al. (1993).

M Classification

M1:   Lower thoracic oesophagus:
       M1a   Metastasis in coeliac lymph nodes
       M1b   Other distant metastasis
       Upper thoracic oesophagus:
       M1a   Metastasis in cervical lymph nodes
       M1b   Other distant metastasis

Justification: In contrast to former data (Japanese Committee for Registration of Esophageal carcinoma 1985) recent observations suggest differences in prognosis between proposed categories M1a and M1b (Kato et al. 1993, Iizuka (1993).

Stomach

T Classification

T1:   T1a   Tumour invades lamina propria (mucosa)
       T1b   Tumour invades submucosa

Justification: ECC: different frequency of lymph node metastasis, different treatment, important as indication for treatment by limited procedures (Inoue et al. 1991).

T2   T2a   Tumor invades muscularis propria
       T2b   Tumor invades subserosa

Justification: ECC: Stomach carcinoma, any type, treated by resection for cure (RO), survival observed, surgical mortality not excluded (Kaplan–Meier):

	Number of patients	2-year survival rate ± standard error (%)	5-year survival rate ± standard error (%)	Median survival time (months)
pT2a	84	74 ± 5	62 ± 6	118.6
pT2b	306	57 ± 3	40 ± 4	36.4

The difference was statistically significant ($p < 0.01$).

An additional argument is the frequency of regional lymph node metastasis: in pT2a, 29/83 (24.9%); and in pT2b, 216/306 (70.6%) ($p < 0.001$).

Siewert and Bollschweiler (1992) observed the following survival in stomach carcinoma, any type, treated by resection for cure (R0), surgical mortality not excluded (Kaplan–Meier):

	Number of patients	2-year survival rate ± standard error (%)	5-year-survival rate ± standard error (%)	Median survival time (months)
pT2a	75	73 ± 7	55 ± 10	94
pT2b	83	51 ± 7	37 ± 8	24

The difference was statistically significant ($p < 0.01$).

An additional argument is the frequency of regional lymph node metastasis: in pT2a, 27/75 (36%); and in pT2b, 61/83 (73.5%) ($p < 0.01$).

Harrison et al. (1992) reported better prognosis for gastric adenocarcinoma limited to the muscularis propria and confirmed this finding by multivariate analysis.

N Classification

N1, N2 a 1–3 nodes involved
        b 4–6 nodes involved
        c > 6 nodes involved

Justification. The correlation between the number of involved regional lymph nodes and 5-year survival has been shown in several publications (Haruyama et al. 1981; Kanabe et al. 1983; Kim and Jung 1987; Shin et al. 1989; Okusa et al. 1990; Stöltzing et al. 1990; Kim et al. 1992). The best discrimination is achieved by the subdivision of Okusa et al. (1990) into 1–3, 4–6 and > 6 nodes:

Number of nodes involved	Number of patients	5-year-survival rate (%)
1–3	85	63
4–6	42	47
> 6	68	29

Colon and Rectum

pT Classification

pT3   pT3a   Minimal: Tumour invades through the muscularis propria into the subserosa or into nonperitonealized pericolic or perirectal tissues, not more than 1 mm beyond the outer border of muscularis propria

pT3b   Slight: Tumour invades through the muscularis propria into the subserosa or into nonperitonealized pericolic or perirectal tissues, more than 1 mm but not more than 5 mm beyond the outer border of muscularis propria

pT3c   Moderate: Tumour invades through the muscularis propria into the subserosa or into nonperitonealized pericolic or perirectal tissues, more than 5 mm but not more than 15 mm beyond the outer border of the muscularis propria

pT3d   Extensive: Tumour invades through the muscularis propria into the subserosa or into nonperitonealized pericolic or perirectal tissues, more than 15 mm beyond outer border of muscularis propria

Justification. The extent of perimuscular invasion seems to influence prognosis, especially in rectum carcinoma, but such reports are still controversial (Fielding et al. 1991). Therefore, further studies are needed.

Krook et al. (1991) subdivided pT3 into microscopic and gross involvement and adherence to adjacent organs.

Cawthorn et al. (1990) reported the following 5-year survival for resected rectum carcinoma patients (any R):

Invasion beyond muscularis propria	Stage II (pNO)	Stage III pN1–3)	Total
⩽ 4 mm	66%	30%	55%
> 4 mm	37%	18%	25%

In the ERCRC and SGCRC studies the perimuscular invasion was subdivided according to histological measurements into ⩽ 5, > 5 to 15 and > 15 mm, in the Swiss Registration Study Colorectal Cancer (SAKK study) (Torhorst 1991) into ⩽ 5 and > 5 mm. The respective unpublished data are as follows:

- SAKK (Torhorst 1991), colon and rectum carcinoma, pN0 only, observed survival 30 months (Kaplan–Meier, surgical mortality not excluded): ⩽ 5 mm ($n = 143$), 90%; > 5 mm ($n = 106$), 62%.
- ERCRC, 1978–1988, radical resection for cure (R0), 5-year survival rates (Kaplan–Meier, surgical mortality not excluded):

Tumour site, pN	Extension of perimuscular invasion (mm)	Number of patients	5-year survival rate ± standard error (%)		
			Observed	Relative	
Rectum	≤ 5	134	75.5 ± 4.8	92 ± 5.8	$p < 0.01$
pN 0	> 5	133	62.2 ± 4.9	75.7 ± 5.9	
Rectum	≤ 5	102	52.8 ± 6.4	63.6 ± 7.7	$p < 0.01$
pN 1–3	> 5	212	37.2 ± 4.2	44.3 ± 4.9	
Colon	≤ 5	106	89.3 ± 4.1	100 – 3.7	n. s.
pN 0	> 5	163	83.1 ± 3.6	100 – 2.5	
Colon	≤ 5	35	53.3 ± 12.5	62.4 ± 13.5	n. s.
pN 1–3	> 5	179	54.3 ± 4.7	67.2 ± 5.8	

– SGCRC; 1984–1986, radical resection for cure (R 0), 5-year survival rates (Kaplan–Meier, surgical mortality not excluded):

Tumour site, pN	Extension of perimuscular invasion (mm)	Number of patients	5-year survival rate ± standard error (%)		
			Observed	Relative	
Rectum	≤ 5	128	58.9 ± 4.8	75.0 ± 6.1	n. s.
pN 0	> 5	115	58.6 ± 5.1	72.1 ± 6.2	
Rectum	≤ 5	76	47.0 ± 6.0	59.7 ± 7.6	$p < 0.05$
pN 1–3	> 5	183	31.9 ± 3.6	38.6 ± 4.3	
Colon	≤ 5	112	70.5 ± 4.7	92.2 ± 6.1	n. s.
pN 0	> 5	232	66.3 ± 3.4	89.2 ± 4.6	
Colon	≤ 5	42	52.4 ± 7.9	65.3 ± 9.9	n. s.
pN 1–3	> 5	201	42.4 ± 3.8	56.2 ± 5.0	

For further investigation a subdivision into 4 subgroups is recommended because of general considerations, although supporting data are not available. For those preferring a simpler subdivision, pT 3a and b as well as pT 3c and d may be combined.

pT 4   pT 4a   Invasion of adjacent organs or structures, without perforation of visceral peritoneum
          pT 4b   Perforation of visceral peritoneum

Justification. Unpublished data of the ERCRC showed the following frequencies of distant metastasis: pT 4a, 66/211 (31.3 %); pT 4b, 107/208 (51.4 %). The prognosis following resection for cure (RO), surgical mortality not excluded, was as follows (Kaplan–Meier).

	Number of patients	5-year survival rate ± standard error (%)		Median survival time (months)
		Observed	Relative	
pT 4a M0	83	49 ± 7	60 ± 9	58.2
pT 4b M0	93	43 ± 8	53 ± 9	46.2
pT 4a M1	13	12 ± 11	14 ± 13	22.7
pT 4b M1	24	0	0	15.5

The differences were not statistically significant.

Unpublished data from the Concord Hospital, Sydney, Australia, show a significant influence in multivariate analyses (Chapuis 1992).

Liver

T Classification

T4   T4a   Multiple tumours in more than one lobe, none more than 2 cm in greatest dimension
    T4b   Multiple tumours in more than one lobe, any more than 2 cm in greatest dimensions
    T4c   Tumour(s) involving a major branch of the portal or hepatic vein(s)
    T4d   Tumour(s) involving adjacent organ(s) (excluding gallbladder)
    T4e   Tumour with perforation of visceral peritoneum

Justification. Japanese report at the UICC TNM Meeting 1989, DSK-TNM.

Gallbladder

T Classification

T3   T3a   Tumour perforates the serosa (visceral peritoneum) or directly invades into liver (extension 2 cm or less) or both
    T3b   Tumour perforates the serosa (visceral peritoneum) or directly invades into one adjacent organ other than liver
T4   T4a   Tumour extends more than 2 cm into liver
    T4b   Tumour extends into two or more adjacent organs (stomach, duodenum, colon, pancreas, omentum, extrahepatic bile ducts, any involvement of liver)

Justification. Preliminary data shows different prognosis for patients with tumour resection (ECC).

Extrahepatic Bile Ducts

T Classification

T3   T3a   Tumour invades gallbladder (no other adjacent structures)

T3b   Tumour invades adjacent structures other than gallbladder (liver, pancreas, duodenum, colon, stomach)

Justification. Different treatment, different prognosis (ECC).

Pancreas

T Classification

T3   T3a   Tumour extends directly to any of the following: stomach, spleen, colon

T3b   Tumour extends directly to adjacent large vessels

Justification. ICC Report 1989, for treatment planning.

N Classification

N1   N1a   Metastasis in a single regional lymph node

N1b   Metastasis in multiple regional lymph nodes

Justification. Different prognosis (Hermanek 1991).

	Number of patients	2-year survival rate ± standard error (%)	5-year survival rate ± standard error (%)	Median survival time (months)
pN1a	12	51 ± 17	30 ± 16	19.5
pN1b	54	18 ± 7	0	6.1

The difference is statistically significant ($p < 0.01$).

Lung Tumours

T Classification

T3   T3a   Atelectasis or obstructive pneumonitis of the entire lung, no other criteria for T3 present

T3b   Other criteria for T3

Justification. Results of German TNM Lung Cancer Study (Bülzebruck et al. 1989).

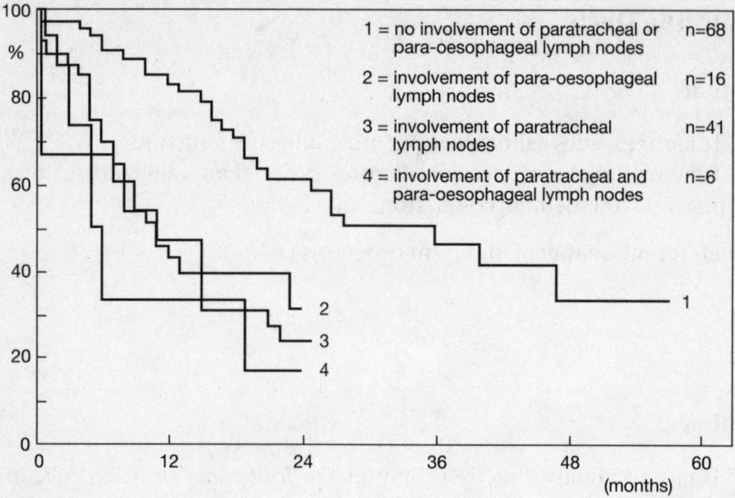

Fig. 26. Prognosis in lung carcinoma following resection in relation to mediastinal lymph node involvement. (From Drings et al. 1992)

T4   T4a   Criteria for T4 excluding b below
       T4b   Invasion of carina or tumour with malignant pleural effusion

Justification. Results of German TNM Lung Cancer Study (Bülzebruck et al. 1989)

N Classification

N2   N2a   Metastasis in ipsilateral mediastinal lymph nodes other than paratracheal and para-oesophageal
       N2b   Metastasis in ipsilateral paratracheal or para-oesophageal lymph nodes

Justification. Different prognosis (Fig. 26), also confirmed by multivariate analysis (Bülzebruck et al. 1991 a, b; Drings et al. 1992).

N3   N3a   Intrathoracic lymph node metastasis only (contralateral mediastinal or contralateral hilar)
       N3b   Scalene or supraclavicular lymph node metastasis

Justification. Different radiotherapy procedures (Hamburg Radiological Centre).

M Classification

M1   M1a   Distant metastasis limited to contralateral lung (intraparenchymal and/or pleura)
       M1b   Other distant metastasis

Justification. For treatment planning, different prognosis, according to unpublished data of Bülzebruck et al. (1992):

	Patients with tumour resection		All patients (± tumour resection)	
	M1a	M1b	M1a	M1b
Number of patients	108	46	341	829
1-year survival (%)	57	29	32	17
3-year survival (%)	28	7	10	3
5-year survival (%)	14	2	5	1
Median survival time (months)	14	6	7	5
	$p < 0.001$		$p < 0.001$	

Tumours of Bone and Soft Tissues

Bone

T Classification

T1, T2   a   Tumour 15 cm or less in greatest dimension
          b   Tumour more than 15 cm in greatest dimension

Justification. Different prognosis according to JJC report 1992 (unpublished data of H. Fukuma).

T2   (i)   Beyond cortex to periosteum
      (ii)   Beyond periosteum to surrounding soft tissues
      (iii)   With extension to major vessels or nerves

Justification. ICC report 1989, for treatment planning.

Soft Tissues

T Classification

T1, T2   a   No involvement of major blood vessels or nerves and, for mediastinal and retroperitoneal tumours, no invasion of adjacent organs
              (i)   intracompartmental
              (ii) extracompartmental
          b   Involvement of major blood vessels or nerves
          c   Invasion of bones or, for mediastinal and retroperitoneal tumours, invasion of adjacent organs

Note. A compartment is defined as an anatomical space bounded by natural barriers to tumour extension such as fascias, ligaments, tendons, tendon sheaths, cortical bone, articular cartilage, joint capsule.

Justification. ICC report 1989, for treatment planning.

Skin Tumours

Carcinoma of Skin

T Classification

T1–3   a   Limited to dermis and 2 mm or less in thickness
         b   Limited to dermis and more than 2 mm but not more than 6 mm in thickness
         c   Invading the subcutis and/or more than 6 mm in thickness
T4   a   6 mm or less in thickness
         b   More than 6 mm in thickness

Justification. This subdivision seems important for treatment planning as it correlates with the risk of regional lymph node metastasis (Breuninger et al. 1988, 1990).

Category	Frequency of regional lymph node metastasis during follow-up of 2–13 years (median 6.5 years) (%)
T1a	0
T1b	4.5
T1c	15–20 [a]
T3c	15–30 [a]
T4a	25–30 [a]
T4b	30–40 [a]

[a] According to histological grade.

Malignant Melanoma of Skin

pT Classification: Ulceration

Any pT   (u–)   No ulceration
           (u+)   Ulceration

Justification. Proposal JJC 1991, different prognosis (Balch et al. 1992).

Consideration of the Clark Level in pT Classification

There are some discussions on the relative prognostic significance of tumour thickness and Clark levels, in particular whether the predominance of tumour thickness still justifies the inclusion of Clark levels in the definition of PT (Garbe et al. 1990;

Häffner et al. 1992; Ketcham et al. 1992; Morton et al. 1993). Some authors are of the opinion that in case of discrepancy between tumour thickness and Clark level, thickness should take precedence in the assignment of pT:

Present pT definitions follow the rule that in discrepancies between tumour thickness and level the pT category is based on the less favourable finding:

Tumour thickness (mm)	Clark level			
	2	3	4	5
≤ 0.75	pT1			
> 0.75–1.50		pT2		
> 1.50–3.00			pT3a	
> 3.00–4.00		pT3b		
> 4.00				pT4a

Proposal for pT definitions following the rule of precedence of tumour thickness:

Tumour thickness (mm)	Clark level			
	2	3	4	5
≤ 0.75		pT1		
> 0.75–1.50		pT2		
> 1.50–3.00		pT3a		
> 3.00-4.00		pT3b		
> 4.00		pT4a		

Example. A melanoma with a thickness of 1.40 mm and level 4 is classified according to the present TNM as pT3a. However, according to the above opinion this tumour should be classified as pT2.

Proposed Ramification of Present pT Classification

For clarification the ECC proposes further studies using the following ramification:

pT2	(i)	≤ 0.75 mm
	(ii)	> 0.75–1.50 mm
pT3a	(i)	≤ 0.75 mm
	(ii)	> 0.75–1.50 mm
	(iii)	> 1.50–3.00 mm
pT4a	(i)	≤ 0.75 mm
	(ii)	> 0.75–1.50 mm
	(iii)	> 1.50–3.00 mm
	(iv)	> 3.00–4.00 mm
	(v)	> 4.00 mm

With this ramification a comparison between the present pT classification and the proposed one is possible.

Conversion Tables

Present	New		New	Present
pT1	pT1		pT1	pT1
				pT2(i)
pT2(i)	pT1			pT3a(i)
pT2(ii)	pT2			pT4a(i)
pT3a(i)	pT1		pT2	pT2(ii)
pT3a(ii)	pT2			pT3a(ii)
pT3a(iii)	pT3a			pT4a(ii)
pT3b	pT3b		pT3a	pT3a(iii)
				pT4a(iii)
pT4a(i)	pT1			
pT4a(ii)	pT2		pT3b	pT3b
pT4a(iii)	pT3a			pT4a(iv)
pT4a(iv)	pT3b			
pT4a(v)	pT4a		pT4a	pT4a(v)

Justification. For comparison between the present pT classification and a possible pT classification based on tumour thickness alone, Garbe (1992) presented survival data of a cooperative study of four German departments of dermatology (Berlin, Münster-Hornheide, Tübingen, Würzburg). The study includes 4830 patients treated between 1970 and 1989.

Adjusted survival rates in relation to the present UICC pT classification and to tumour thickness alone (calculation according to Cutler–Ederer) where as follows:

Patient groups	Number of patients	Adjusted survival rate ± standard error (%)	
		5 years	10 years
pT1	825	99.1 ± 0.5	96.9 ± 1.5
pT2	1414	95.5 ± 0.7	93.5 ± 1.0
pT3a	1607	84.6 ± 1.1	75.5 ± 1.7[a]
pT3b	389	69.2 ± 2.7	60.5 ± 3.7
pT4a	595	58.4 ± 2.5	46.1 ± 3.3
≤ 0.75 mm	1471	98.4 ± 0.4	97.2 ± 0.9
0.76–1.50 mm	1282	93.8 ± 0.8	90.1 ± 1.3
1.51–3.00 mm	1114	80.9 ± 1.4	69.2 ± 2.2[a]
3.01–4.00 mm	424	68.7 ± 2.6	60.6 ± 3.4
> 4.00 mm	539	57.2 ± 2.6	43.5 ± 3.7

[a] Significantly different: $p < 0.01$

Adjusted survival in relation to pT with ramification according to tumour thickness, as proposed above (p. 129), was as follows:

Patient groups	Number of patients	Adjusted survival (%) rate ± standard error		Significance
		5 years	10 years	
pT2	(i)	594	97.5 ± 0.8	97.1 ± 1.0	
	(ii)	820	94.2 ± 0.1	91.3 ± 1.5	$p = 0.016$
pT3a	(i)	52	97.4 ± 2.6	97.4 ± 2.6	
	(ii)	461	92.9 ± 1.4	88.7 ± 2.2	
	(iii)	1984	80.9 ± 1.4	69.2 ± 2.2	$p < 0.0001$
pT4a	(ii)	1	100	100	
	(iii)	20	84.4 ± 10.3	84.4 ± 10.3	
	(iv)	35	63.4 ± 8.9	57.6 ± 9.8	
	(v)	539	57.2 ± 2.6	43.5 ± 3.7	n. s.

The data can be summarized as follows:

- When comparing the categories of the present pT classification with the corresponding categories considering tumour thickness alone, a significant difference between pT3a and ≤ 1.50–3.00 is found, while the other corresponding categories show no difference.
- In the classification based on thickness alone more patients with excellent survival chances are identified: pT1 and pT2, 2239 (46.4%) versus 2753 (57.0%).
- By ramification of the present pT categories according to tumour thickness, significant differences in survival could be observed within the categories pT2 and pT3a, namely in pT2 better survival for patients with tumour thickness ≤ 0.75 and in pT3a more favourable prognosis for tumour thickness ≤ 1.50 mm. The same trend is seen in pT3a, but the differences are not significant.

The data allow the following preliminary interpretation: About 30% of patients classified pT3a (corresponding to about 10% of the total) have an excellent prognosis with more than 90% survival. This is valid for patients with tumour thickness of 1.50 mm or less. These patients cannot be identified by the present TNM classification. Therefore, the data support a pT classification based on tumour thickness alone. However, confirmation by calculation of nonadjusted observed and relative survival and by data from other institutions is needed. In contrast, recently the importance of both Clark level and tumour thickness was demonstrated by multivariate analysis (Morton et al. 1993).

N Classification

Number of Involved Regional Lymph Nodes

N1   N1a   Single node involved
      N1b   2–4 nodes involved
      N1c   More than 4 nodes involved

Justification. DSK-TNM proposal, different prognosis (Balch et al. 1992; Drepper et al. 1993; Hohenberger et al. 1993).

Size of Involved Regional Lymph Nodes

pN1   pN1(i)   Only micrometastasis (none larger than 0.2 cm)
       pN1(ii)   Metastasis to regional lymph nodes, at least one more than 0.2 cm
                  and all 0.4 cm or less in greatest dimension
       pN1(iii)   Metastasis to regional lymph nodes, at least one more than 0.4 cm
                  and all 3 cm or less in greatest dimension

Justification. Different prognosis (Hermanek 1987; Drepper et al. 1993).

Breast Tumours

T Classification

T1–3   (i)   Without invasion of the underlying fascia and pectoral muscles
        (ii)   With invasion of the underlying fascia and pectoral muscles

Justification. ICC report 1989, for treatment planning.

Satellites

The presence of additional multiple separate microscopic satellites within the breast may be indicated by the addition of "sat" in parentheses.

Justification. Unpublished data of K. Prechtel, Starnberg, FRG, show a trend to an increased frequency of regional lymph node metastasis in case of such satellites:

Tumour size	Satellites	*n*	Regional lymph nodes metastasis *(n)*	(%)
≤ 20 mm	No	164	48	29
	Yes	31	12	39
21–40 mm	No	170	87	51
	Yes	24	15	63

N Classification

N2   N2a   Nodes fixed to one another
      N2b   Nodes fixed to other structures

Justification. ICC report 1989, for treatment planning.

M Classification

M1   M1a   Metastasis in supraclavicular lymph nodes (ipsi- and/or contralateral) only
       M1b   Other distant metastasis

Justification. General considerations, for treatment planning (DSK-TNM).

Gynaecological Tumours

Cervix Uteri

T Classification

T1a2   (i)   Tumour with invasive component 3 mm or less in depth, taken from the base of the epithelium, *and* 7 mm or less in horizontal spread
      (ii)   Tumour with invasive component more than 3 mm but not more than 5 mm in depth, taken from the base of the epithelium, *and* 7 mm or less in horizontal spread

Justification. JJC 1991, for comparison with the classification generally used in Japan.

N Classification

N1   N1a   Metastasis in 1–2 regional lymph nodes below the common iliac artery
       N1b   Metastasis in 3 or more regional lymph nodes below the common iliac artery
       N1c   Metastasis in any lymph node along the common iliac artery

Justification. Dr. Dunst, Erlangen, for treatment planning. Also, data from the literature show the following recurrence rates:

- pN1a, 62 % or 81 % (Alvarez et al. 1989; Shiromizu et al. 1988)
- pN1b, 34 % or 29 % (Alvarez et al. 1989; Shiromizu et al. 1988)

The 5-year survival was found to be

- 1–3 nodes involved, 60 % (Piver and Chung 1975)
- 4 or more nodes involved, 38 % (Piver and Chung 1975)
- pN1a,b 53 % or 63 % (Hsu et al. 1972; Kjorstad et al. 1984)
- pN1c, 21 % or 30 % (Hsu et al. 1972; Kjorstad et al. 1984)

In one investigation (Alvarez et al. 1989) the number of involved nodes was found to be an independent prognostic factor by multivariate analysis. The respective classes were 1–2 versus 3 or more nodes involved.

M Classification

M1   M1a   Distant metastasis in para-aortic lymph nodes below the diaphragm only

M1b   Distant metastasis in other sites

Justification. The 5-year survival rate in patients with para-aortic node metastases only treated by radiotherapy was 29 % (Nori et al. 1985).

Urological Tumours

Penis

T Classification

T1, T2   a   Tumour 2 cm or less in greatest dimension

b   Tumour more than 2 cm but not more than 5 cm in greatest dimension

c   Tumour more than 5 cm in greatest dimension

Justification. For treatment planning and for comparability with the classification of Maiche and Pyrhönen (1990).

Prostate

T Classification

T4a   (i)   Tumour invades bladder neck

(ii)   Tumour invades external sphincter

(iii)   (i) and (ii)

(iv)   Tumour invades rectum

T4b   (i)   Tumour invades levator muscles

(ii)   Tumour is fixed to pelvic wall

(iii)   (i) and (ii)

Justification. Insufficient information on prognostic significance, therapeutic implications (Schröder et al. 1992).

pN Classification

pN 1   a   Metastasis in a single lymph node, 0.2 cm or less in greatest dimension
         b   Metastasis in a single lymph node, more than 0.2 cm but not more than 2 cm in greatest dimension
pN 2a   a   Metastasis in multiple lymph nodes, none more than 0.2 cm in greatest dimension
         b   Metastasis in a single lymph node, more than 2 cm but not more than 5 cm in greatest dimension
         c   Metastasis in multiple lymph nodes, at least one more than 0.2 cm and none more than 5 m in greatest dimension

Justification. Significance of micrometastasis not sufficiently clear, recommendation of Schröder et al. (1992).

M Classification

M 1b   (i)   Metastasis in bone(s), 1–5 foci
         (ii)   Metastasis in bone(s), > 5–20 foci
         (iii)   Metastasis in bone(s), more than 20 foci or diffuse metastatic involvement

Justification. Different prognosis (Soloway et al. 1987), recommendation of Schröder et al. (1992). The 2-year survival rates were: M 1b(i), 95 %; M 1b(ii), 75 %; M 1b(iii), 50 % (Soloway et al. 1987).

Testis

pT Classification

pT 1   pT 1a   Tumour limited to testis
         pT 1b   Tumour invades the rete testis

Justification. Different prognosis, according to Freedman et al. (1987).

pT 2   pT 2a   Tumour invades beyond tunica albuginea
         pT 2b   Tumour invades into epididymis

Justification. Different prognosis, according to Hoskin et al. (1986) and Freedman et al. (1987).

N Classification

N3   N3a   Metastasis in a lymph node, more than 5 cm but not more than 10 cm in greatest dimension

N3b   Metastasis in a lymph node, more than 10 cm in greatest dimension

Justification. Proposal of Pirtoli et al. (1988), because of different prognosis and treatment in seminoma.

Kidney

T Classification

T2   T2a   Tumour more than 2.5 cm but not more than 5 cm in greatest dimension, limited to the kidney

T2b   Tumour more than 5 cm but not more than 7.5 cm in greatest dimension, limited to the kidney

T2c   Tumour more than 7.5 cm but not more than 10 cm in greatest dimension, limited to the kidney

T2d   Tumour more than 10 cm in greatest dimension, limited to the kidney

Justification. Different prognosis according to size (Hermanek and Schrott 1990; Guinan et al. 1992); for separate analysis of patients treated by partial nephrectomy.

T1–3a   (i)   Without microscopic venous invasion
         (ii)   With microscopic venous invasion

Justification. Different prognosis (Höhn and Hermanek 1983; Hermanek and Schrott 1990).

Ophthalmic Tumours

Retinoblastoma

T Classification

T1   T1a   Macula not involved
      T1b   Macula involved
T2   T2a   Macula not involved
      T2b   Macula involved

Justification. Important for evaluation of visual results after treatment (Migdal 1983; Schipper et al. 1985; Kock et al. 1986; Monge et al. 1986).

Paediatric Tumours

Neuroblastoma

M Classification

M 1   M 1 a   Distant metastasis to bone marrow, skin and/or liver
        M 1 b   Other distant metastasis

Justification. In neuroblastoma, the prognosis of patients with distant metastasis depends on the site of metastasis (Evans et al. 1971; Carlsen et al. 1986; Nakagawara et al. 1991).

References

Alajmo K, Antonelli A, Carrogio A, Cervellera G, Miani P, Molinari R, Serafini I (1988) TNM 1987: Problematiche correlate alle classificazione del tumori della testa e del colle. Acta Otorhinolaryngol Ital 8: 321–370

Alvarez RD, Soong SJ, Kinney WK, Reid GC, Schray MF, Podratz KC, Morley GW, Shingleton HM (1989) Identification of prognostic factors and risk groups in patients found to have nodal metastasis at the time of radical hysterectomy for early-stage squamous carcinoma of the cervix. Gynecol Oncol 35: 130–135

Balch CM, Soong SJ, Shaw HM, Urist MM, McCarthy WH (1992) An analysis of prognostic factors in 8500 patients with cutaneous melanoma. In: Balch CM, Houghton AN, Milton GW, Sober AJ, Soong SJ (eds) Cutaneous melanoma, 2nd edn. Lippincott, Philadelphia

Bittesini L, Dei Tos AP, Della Libera D, Carlon G (1991) Proposta per une classificazione pT anatomiamente orientata. In: Serafini I (ed) Il carcinoma glottico a sottoglottico. Piccin Nuova Libraria, Padova, pp 145–147

Breuninger H, Langer B, Rassner G (1988) Untersuchungen zur Prognosebestimmung des spinozellulären Karzinoms der Haut und Unterlippe an Hand des TNM-Systems und zusätzlicher Parameter. Hautart 39: 430–434

Breuninger H, Black B, Rassner G (1990) Microstaging of squamous cell carcinoma. Am J Clin Pathol 94: 624–627

Bülzebruck H, Probst G, Vogt-Moykopf I (1989) Validierung des TNM-Systems für das Bronchialkarzinom: Güte der klinischen Klassifikation, Wertigkeit diagnostischer Verfahren und prognostische Relevanz. Z Herz Thorax Gefäßchirur 3: 195–208

Bülzebruck H, Krysa S, Bauer E, Probst G, Drings P, Vogt-Moykopf I (1991 a) Validation of the TNM classification (4th ed) for lung cancer – first results of a prospective study of 1086 patients with surgical treatment. Eur J Cardiothorac Surg 5: 356–362

Bülzebruck H, Drings P, Kayser K, Schulz V, Tuengertal S, Vogt-Moykopf I (1991 b) Classification of lung cancer: first experience with the new TNM Classification (4th edition). Eur Respir J 4: 1197–1206

Bülzebruck H, Drings P, Vogt-Moykopf I (1992) Personal communication

Calearo C (1991) L'attualità classificativa e la sua problematica a livello glottico. In: Serafini I (ed) Il carcinoma glottico e sottoglottico. Piccin Nuova Libraria, Padova, pp 137–144

Carlsen NLT, Christensen IJ, Schroeder H, Bro PV, Hesselbjerg U, Jensen KB, Nielsen OH (1986) Prognostic value of different staging systems in neuroblastomas and completeness of tumor excision. Arch Dis Child 61: 832–842

Cawthorn SJ, Parums DV, Gibbs NM, A'Hern RP, Caffarey SM, Broughton CIM, Marks CG (1990) Extent of mesorectal spread and involvement of lateral resection margin as prognostic factors after surgery for rectal cancer. Lancet i: 1055–1059

Ceci G, Franciosi V, Nizzoli R, de Kisi V, Lottici R, Boni C, di Blasio B, Passalacqua R, Guazzi A, Cocconi G (1988) The value of bone marrow biopsy in breast cancer at time of diagnosis. Cancer 61: 96–98

Chapuis PH (1992) Personal communication

Cote R, Rosen PP, Hakes TB, Sedira M, Bazinet M, Kinne DW, Old LJ, Osborne MP (1988) Monoclonal antibodies detect occult breast carcinoma metastases in the bone marrow of patients with early stage disease. Am J Surg Pathol 12: 333–340

Cote RJ, Rosen PP, Leser ML, Old LJ, Osborne MP (1991) Monoclonal antibodies detect occult breast carcinoma metastases in the bone marrow of patients with early stage disease. J Clin Oncol 9: 1749–1756

Dralle H (1992) Personal communication

Dralle H, Damm I, Scheumann GFW, Kotzerke J, Kupsch E, Geerlings H, Pichlmayr R (1993) Compartment-oriented microdissection of regional lymph nodes in medullary thyroid carcinoma. World J Surg (in press)

Drepper H, Bieß B, Hofherr B, Hundeiker M, Lippold A, Otto F, Padberg G, Peters A, Wiebelt H (1992) The prognosis of patients with stage III melanoma. Prospective long-term study on 286 patients of the Fachklinik Hornheide. Cancer 71: 1239–1246

Drings P, Vogt-Moykopf I, Bültzebruck H (1992) Personal communication

Endo M, Takeshita K, Yoshino K (1988) Oesophagoscopy for the diagnosis of superficial oesophageal cancer. Surg Endosc 2: 205–208

Evans AE, d'Angio GJ, Randolph J (1971) A proposed staging for children with neuroblastoma. Cancer 27: 374–378

Fielding LP, Arsenault PA, Chapuis PH, Dent O, Gatright B, Hardcastle JD, Hermanek P, Jass JR, Newland RC (1991) Clinicopathological staging for colorectal cancer: An International Documentation System (IDS) and an International Comprehensive Anatomical Terminology (ICAT). J Gastroenterol Hepatol 6: 325–344

Fleischer I (1977) Morphologische Untersuchungen an subglottischen Kehlkopfcarcinomen. Inaugural Dissertation, University of Marburg, FRG

Freedman LS, Parkinson MC, Jones WG, Oliver RTD, Peckham MJ, Read G, Newlands ES, Williams CJ (1987) Histopathology in the prediction of relapse of patients with stage I testicular teratoma treated by orchiectomy alone. Lancet ii: 294–298

Garbe C, Büttner P, Bertz J, Burg G, d'Hoedt B, Drepper H, Guggenmoos-Holzmann I, Lechner W, Lippold A, Orfanos CE, Peters A, Rassner G, Schwermann M, Stadler R, Stroebel W (1990) Prognose des primären malignen Melanoms. Eine multizentrische Studie an 5093 Patienten. In: Orfanos CE, Garbe C (eds) Das maligne Melanom der Haut. Zuckschwerdt, Munich

Garbe C (1992) Personal communication

Glanz HK (1984) Carcinoma of the larynx. Growth, p-classification and grading of squamous cell carcinoma of the vocal cords. Adv Oto-rhinolaryngol 32: 1–123

Glanz H (1986) pT-Klassifikation der Larynxkarzinome. In: Hermanek P (ed) Bedeutung des TNM-Systems für die klinische Onkologie. Zuckschwerdt, Munich

Glanz HK (1992) Personal communication

Glanz HK, Eichhorn T (1989) Prognoserelevante pathohistologische Klassifikation von Halslymphknotenmetastasen (pN) laryngologischer Karzinome. HNO 37: 481–484

Glanz HK, Popella C (1993) Prognoserelevanz der pTpN-Klassifikation von Larynxkarzinomen und ihre Bedeutung für die Verbesserung der TN-Klassifikation. (in preparation)

Guinan P, Targonski P, Frank W, Rubenstein M (1992) Unpublished data reported to the UICC TNM Committee

Häffner AC, Garbe C, Burg G, Büttner P, Orfanos CE, Rassner G (1992) The prognosis of primary and metastasising melanoma. An evaluation of the TNM classification in 2495 patients. Br J Cancer 66, 856–861

Harrison JC, Dean PJ, van der Zwaag R, el-Zeky F, Wruble ID (1991) Adenocarcinoma of the stomach with invasion limited to the muscularis propria. Hum Pathol 22: 111–117

Haruyama K (1981) Quantitative statistical studies on lymph node metastasis of gastric carcinoma, with reference to its relationship with primary lesion and prognosis. J Jap Surg Soc 82: 612–621

Hausamen JE (1988) Tasks and objectives of the German-Austrian-Swiss Working Group on Tumours in the Maxillo-Facial Region (DOESAK). Int J Oral Maxillofac Surg 17: 264–266

Hermanek P (1987) Lymphogene Metastasierung des malignen Melanoms, Häufigkeit, Klassifikation und prognostische Bedeutung. Acta Chir Austr 19: 249–250

Hermanek P (1991) Staging of exocrine pancreatic carcinoma. Eur J Surg Oncol 17: 167–172

Hermanek P, Schrott KM (1990) Evaluation of the new tumor, nodes and metastasis classification of renal cell carcinoma. J Urol 144: 238–244

Hirayama K, Mori S (1990) Prognostic factors in early esophageal cancer. Gan To Kagaku Ryoho 17: 37–45

Ho JHC (1970) The natural history and treatment of nasopharyngeal carcinoma. In: Lee-Clark R, Cumley RW, McCay JE, Copeland M (eds) Proceedings of the X international cancer congress, vol 4. Yearbook, Chicago

Ho JHC (1978 a) An epidemiologic and clinical study of nasopharyngeal carcinoma. Int J Radiat Oncol Biol Phys 4: 183–188

Ho JHC (1978 b) Stage classification of nasopharyngeal carcinoma. A review. In: de Thé G, Ito Y (eds) Nasopharyngeal carcinoma. Etiology and Control. IARC, Lyon, pp 99–113 (Scientific publication no 20)

Höhn W, Hermanek P (1983) Invasion of veins in renal cell carcinoma – frequency, correlation and prognosis. Eur Urol 9: 276–280

Hohenberger W, Göhl J, Kessler C (1993) Prophylaktische und therapeutische Lymphknotendissektion bei malignem Melanom. Chirurg BDC 32: 7–9

Hoskin P, Dilly S, Easton D, Horwich A, Hendry W, Peckham MJ (1986) Prognostic factors in stage I non-seminomatous germ-cell testicular tumors managed by orchiectomy and surveillance. J Clin Oncol 4: 1031–1036

Howaldt HJ, Pitz H, Frenz M (1991) Aufbau und erste Ergebnisse eines Registers für Malignome im Mund-, Kiefer- und Gesichtsbereich. In: van Eimeren W, Überla K, Ulm K (eds) Gesundheit und Umwelt. Springer, Berlin Heidelberg New York

Howaldt HJ, Frenz M, Pitz H (1992) Proposals for a modified T classification for oral cancer. J Cranio-Maxillo-Facial Surg 21: 96–101

Hsu CT, Cheng YS, Su SC (1972) Prognosis of uterine cervical cancer with extensive lymph node metastases. Am J Obstet Gynecal 114: 954–962

Iizuka T (1993) The fourth edition of the UICC TNM classification of esophageal carcinoma and its relevance for comparison of international data. In: Sato T, Iizuka T (eds) Color atlas of surgical anatomy for esophageal cancer. Springer, Tokyo Berlin Heidelberg New York

Inoue K, Tobe T, Kan N, Nio Y, Sakai M, Takeuchi E, Sugiyama T (1991) Problems in the definition and treatment of early gastric cancer. Br J Surg 78: 818–821

Japanese Committee for Registration of Esophageal Carcinoma (1985) A proposal for a new TNM classification of esophageal carcinoma. Jpn J Clin Oncol 14: 625–636

Jauch KW, Heiss M, Funke I, Grützner V, Pantel K, Riethmüller G, Schildberg FW (1992) Tumor cell spread to bone marrow in gastric cancer. J Cancer Res Clin Oncol 118 (Suppl R): 23

Kanabe S, Omori Y, Honda I (1983) Numerical analysis of lymph node metastasis of gastric carcinoma. Jap J Gastric Surg 16: 1766–1771

Karim ABMF, Kralendonk JH, Njo KH, Tabak JM, Gort G (1990) A critical look at the TNM classification for laryngeal carcinoma. Cancer 65: 1918–1922

Kato H, Tachimori Y, Watanabe H, Iizuka T (1993) Evaluation of the new (1987) TNM classification for thoracic esophageal tumors. Int J Cancer 53: 220–223

Ketcham AS, Moffat FL, Balch CM (1992) Classification and staging. In: Balch CM, Houghton AN, Milton GW, Sober AJ, Soong SJ (eds) Cutaneous melanoma, 2nd edn. Lippincott, Philadelphia

Kim JP, Jung SE (1987) Patients with gastric cancer and their prognosis in accordance with number of lymph node metastases. Scand J Gastroenterol 22, Suppl 133: 33–35

Kim JP, Yang H-K, Oh ST (1992) Is the new UICC staging system of gastric cancer reasonable? (Comparison of 5-year survival rate of gastric cancer by old and new UICC stage classification). Surgical Oncology 1: 209–213

Kirk SJ, Cooper GG, Hoper M, Watt PCH, Roy AD, Odling-Smee W (1990) The prognostic significance of marrow micrometastases in women with early breast cancer. Eur J Surg Oncol 16: 481–485

Kjorstadt KE, Kolbenstvedt A, Strickert T (1984) The value of complete lymphadenectomy in radical treatment of cancer of the cervix, stage I_B. Cancer 54: 2215–2219

Kleinsasser O (1986) TNM-Klassifikation der Larynxkarzinome. In: Hermanek P (ed) Bedeutung des TNM-Systems für die klinische Onkologie. Zuckschwerdt, Munich

Kleinsasser O (1992) Revision of classification of laryngeal cancer, is it long overdue? (Proposals for an improved TN-classification). J Laryngol Otol 106: 197–204

Kleinsasser O, Glanz H (1992) Personal communication (to be published)

Kock E, Rosengren B, Tengroth B, Trampe E (1986) Retinoblastoma treated with a ^{60}Co applicator. Radiother Oncol 7: 19–26

Krook J, Moertel C, Gunderson LL, Wieand HS, Collins RT, Beart RW, Kubista TP, Poon MA, Meyers WC, Maillard JA, Twito DI, Morton RF, Veeder MH, Witzig TE, Cha S, Vidyarthi SC (1991) Effective surgical adjuvant therapy for high-risk rectal carcinoma. N Engl J Med 324: 709–715

Lindemann F, Schlimok G, Dirschedl P, Witte J, Riethmüller G (1992) Prognostic significance of micrometastatic tumour cells in bone marrow of colorectal cancer patients. Lancet 340: 685–689

Maiche AG, Pyrhönen S (1990) Clinical staging of cancer of the penis: by size? by localization? or by depth of infiltration? Eur Urol 18: 16–22

Mansi JL, Berger U, Easton D, McDonnell T, Redding WH, Gazet JC, McKinna A, Powles TJ, Coombes RC (1987) Micrometastases in bone marrow in patients with primary breast cancer; evaluation as an early predictor of bone metastasis. BMJ 295: 1093–1096

Mansi JL, Berger U, McDonnell T, Pople A, Rayter Z, Gazet MC, Coombes RC (1989) The fate of bone marrow micrometastases in patients with primary breast cancer. J Clin Oncol 7: 445–449

Matsubara T, Nakajima T, Nishi M, Kaise T, Ishiguro M (1993) Which is the superior staging system for evaluating the degree of lymphatic extension in cancer of the thoracic esophagus. Abstracts UICC Kyoto International Symposion on Recent Advances in Management of Digestive Cancer. p 106

Meyer-Breiting E (1990) Überlegungen und Untersuchungen zur Klassifikation glottischer Karzinome. Laryngol Rhinol Otol 69: 6–12

Meyer-Breiting E, Bettinger R (1991) Zur T-Klassifikation supraglottischer Tumoren. Arch ORL Suppl II: 180–190

Migdal C (1983) Bilateral retinoblastoma: the prognosis for vision. Br J Ophthalmol 67: 592–595

Molinari R (1990) Clinical classification of laryngeal carcinoma: proposal for a new method of classification. Acta Otorhinolaryngol Ital 10: 579–591

Molino A, Colombatti M, Bonetti F, Zardini M, Pasini F, Perini A, Pelosi G, Tridente G, Veneri G, Cetto GL (1991) A comparative analysis of three different techniques for the detection of breast cancer cells in bone marrow. Cancer 67: 1033–1036

Monge OR, Flage T, Hatlevoll R, Vermund H (1986) Sight-saving therapy in retinoblastoma. Experience with external megavoltage radiotherapy. Acta Ophthalmol 64: 414–420

Morton DL, Davtyan DG, Wanek LA, Foshag LJ, Cochran AJ (1993) Multivariate analysis of the relationship between survival and the microstage of primary melanoma by Clark level and Breslow thickness. Cancer 71: 3737–3743

Nakagawara A, Morita K, Okabe I, Uchino J, Ohi R, Iwafuchi M, Matsuyama S, Nagashima K, Takahashi H, Nakajo T, Hirai Y, Tsuchida Y, Saeki M, Yokoyama J, Nishi T, Okamoto E, Suita S (1991) Proposal and assessment of Japanese tumor node metastasis postsurgical histopathological staging system for neuroblastoma based on an analysis of 495 cases. Jap J Clin Oncol 21: 1–7

Nori D, Valentine E, Hilaris BS (1989) The role of paraaortic node irradiation in the treatment of cancer of the cervix. Int J Radiat Oncol Biol Phys 11: 1469–1473

Okusa T, Nakane Y, Boku T, Takada H, Yamamura M, Hioki K, Yomemoto M (1990) Quantitative analysis of nodal involvement with respect to survival rate after gastrectomy for carcinoma. Surg Gynecol Obstet 170: 488–494

Pirtoli L, Cionini L, Tucci Z (1988) Radiation therapy and chemotherapy in the management of testicular seminoma: a review. Chemotherapia 7: 63–70

Piver MS, Chung WS (1975) Prognostic significance of cervical lesion size and pelvic node metastases in cervical carcinoma. Obstet Gynecol 46: 507–510

Platz H, Fried R, Hudec M (1986) Prognoses of oral cavity carcinomas. Hansen, Munich

Popella C, Glanz H, Kleinsasser O (1991) Prognoserelevanz der pTpN-Klassifikation von Larynxkarzinomen und ihre Bedeutung für die Verbesserung der TN-Klassifikation. Acta Otorhinolaryngol Suppl IIS: 188–189

Roder JD, Busch R, Stein HJ, Fink U, Siewert JR (1993) Prognostic factors in patients with squamous cell cancer of the esophagus undergoing transthoracic en bloc resection. In: Nabeya K, Hanacka T (eds) Diseases of the esophagus. Springer, Tokyo (in press)

Salvadori B, Squicciarini P, Rovini D (1990) Use of monoclonal antibody MBr1 to detect micrometastases in bone marrow specimens of breast cancer patients. Eur J Cancer 26: 865–866

Schipper J, Tan KEWP, van Peperzeel HA (1985) Treatment of retinoblastoma by precision megavoltage radiation therapy. Radiother Oncol 3: 97–115

Schlimok G, Funke I, Bock B, Schweiberer B, Witte J, Riethmüller G (1990) Epithelial tumor cells in bone marrow of patients with colorectal cancer: immunocytochemical detection, phenotypic characterization, and prognostic significance. J Clin Oncol 8: 831–837

Schlimok G, Funke I, Pantel K, Strobel F, Lindemann F, Witte J, Riethmüller G (1991) Micrometastatic tumour cells in bone marrow of patients with gastric cancer: methodological aspects of detection and prognostic significance. Eur J Cancer 27: 1461–1465

Schlimok G, Lindemann F, Witte J, Riethmüller G (1992) Prognostic significance of bone marrow micrometastasis in gastrointestinal cancer. J Cancer Res Clin Oncol 118 (Suppl R): 24

Schröder FH, Hermanek P, Denis L, Fair WR, Gospodarowicz MK, Pavone-Macaluso M (1992) The TNM classification of prostate cancer. Prostate Suppl 4: 129–138

Shiromizu K, Matsuzawa M, Takahashi M, Ishihara O (1985) Is postoperative radiotherapy or maintenance chemotherapy necessary for carcinoma of the uterine cervix? Br J Obstet Gynaecol 95: 503–506

Shiu MH, Perrotti M, Brennan MF (1989) Adenocarcinoma of the stomach: a multivariate analysis of clinical, pathologic and treatment factors. Hepatogastroenterol 36: 7–12

Siewert JR (1992) Personal communication

Siewert JR, Bollschweiler E (1992) Personal communication

Soloway MS, Hardeman SW, Hickey DP, Todd BB, Soloway SM, Moinuddin M (1987) Simple grading systems for bone scans correlates with survival for patients with stage D2 prostate cancer. J Urol 137: 359A

Steiner W, Ambrosch P (1992) Personal communication

Steiner W, Ambrosch P (1993) A proposal for a modified T classification of head and neck tumors. Otorhinolaryngologica nova (in press)

Stöltzing H, Ohmann C, Thon K (1990) Prognostische Faktoren beim Magenkarzinom. In: Delbrück H (ed) Krebsnachsorge und Rehabilitation, vol 3, Magenkarzinom. Zuckschwerdt, Munich

Tajiri H (1992) Current status of endoscopic ultrasonography and laser palliation on carcinoma of the esophagus. Abstract, international conference on biology and treatment of gastrointestinal malignancies, 4–7 February 1992, Frankfurt, FRG

Torhorst I (1992) Personal communication

Wolfensberger M (1992) Using Cox's proportional hazards model for prognostication in carcinoma of the upper aero-digestive tract. Acta Otolaryngol (Stockh) 112: 376–382

Yoshinaka H, Shimazu H, Fukumoto T, Baba M (1991) Superficial esophageal carcinoma: a clinicopathological review of 59 cases. Am J Gastroenterol 86: 1413–1418

Printing: Saladruck, Berlin
Binding: Buchbinderei Lüderitz & Bauer, Berlin